A Salamander's Tale

A SALAMANDER'S TALE

*My Story of Regeneration—Surviving
30 Years with Prostate Cancer*

PAUL STEINBERG, MD

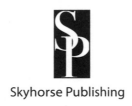

Skyhorse Publishing

Skyhorse Publishing books may be purchased in bulk at special discounts for sales promotion, corporate gifts, fund-raising, or educational purposes. Special editions can also be created to specifications. For details, contact the Special Sales Department, Skyhorse Publishing, 307 West 36th Street, 11th Floor, New York, NY 10018 or info@skyhorsepublishing.com.

Skyhorse® and Skyhorse Publishing® are registered trademarks of Skyhorse Publishing, Inc.®, a Delaware corporation.

www.skyhorsepublishing.com

10 9 8 7 6 5 4 3 2 1

Library of Congress Cataloging-in-Publication Data is available on file.

Print ISBN: 978-1-63220-569-8
Ebook ISBN: 978-1-63220-953-5

Printed in the United States of America

To Helen—Exclamation points cannot fully exclaim and explain your wonders

To Arielle and Miritte and my friends and family—all of whom have bolstered my respirations and aspirations, not to mention giving me some modicum of inspiration

CONTENTS

"Create dangerously, for people who read dangerously . . . Writing, knowing in part that no matter how trivial your words may seem, someday, somewhere, someone may risk his or her life to read them."

—Edwidge Danticant

Prologue

The punishment: the chopping off of my balls, a literal castration. The crime: none, at least none I am aware of. I am not a rapist, let alone a serial rapist. I am not a pedophile. I am not a sex addict. Yes, I do enjoy sex. I am not the greatest lover but I am not the worst. I am good enough.

It is December 1989 and this self-appointed executioner of my love life is talking to me over the phone from New York City. I am in Washington, DC. He is telling me what any self-respecting man would dread to hear: "You need to have your testicles removed. It will save your life. You will die a quick and painful death if you do not undergo a castration." But, wait—what about my very essence, my very spirit as a man, as a human being? Is this a new concept—cut off your balls to save your face?

Your testicles or your life. Not unlike the choice given to Jack Benny by a mugger. "Your money or your life," shouted the mugger to the notoriously cheapskate comedian. Benny stood there paralyzed, unable to choose. Likewise my own paralysis: Doesn't existence lay too much on us? Can existence burden us with any more stark a choice?

I can easily imagine the potential executioners of my orgasms sitting at rounds at a hospital in Manhattan discussing my case. "The patient is a forty-one-year-old white married male psychiatrist living in Washington, DC. He was diagnosed with prostate cancer five years ago and underwent a radical prostatectomy here at our hospital on October 5, 1984. We thought we got it all, every bit of cancerous tissue. To be on the safe side, we had the patient go through six weeks of radiation to the prostate bed in order to eliminate any remaining cancer cells in that area. Unfortunately, there is evidence the cancer has returned. A new test, the 'prostate-specific antigen,' available at this hospital for the past eighteen months, has shown a gradual rise, from 0.6 in 1988 to 2.1 this December. The only source of this antigen has to be cancer cells since his prostate has been completely removed. In a relatively young man like this, with a terribly aggressive disease, the only option is castration. As all of you in this room know, testosterone fuels the growth of these prostate cancer cells. It is urgent and essential that we eliminate all testosterone from this man's body as quickly as possible, and the most expeditious way to do so is by surgical castration."

Over my dead body. Those facts do not tell the full story. They leave out a ton of desire. Where are the yearnings, the struggles and strivings in this doctorly narrative? Where is the mere mention of the orgasm?

Yes, the orgasm. Can there be any more pleasurable experience in a man's or woman's life? Admittedly food and other pleasures can approach the orgasmic, but there is nothing like the real thing. Lust, libido, orgasm: The gods have set it up so that our most vital function—procreation, the survival of the species, the passing on of our genes—is suffused with the most unsubtle of pleasures. As if our instinct to replicate ourselves were not enough, the gods lured us with the promise of an exultant explosion of ecstasy, a momentary pleasure certainly, but one that, with the prospect of repeated paroxysms, can give us a self-assuredness that lasts a seeming lifetime.

Back in the early and mid-twentieth century, the German psychiatrist Wilhelm Reich claimed that without the orgasm, we would all get cancer and would shrivel up and die. On some level this former protégé of Sigmund Freud was simply trying to overcome the sexual repressiveness of Europe and the United States in the nineteenth and early twentieth centuries. Accused of fraud for the promotion of his seemingly useless orgone box, Reich was even willing to go to prison. In fact, he died in the Lewisburg, Pennsylvania, penitentiary attempting to promote the worth of the orgasm.

So here I was, facing the executioner of my orgasms. Although he delivered my sentence in a somber tone, I could not help but wonder how much unacknowledged sadism was involved in this pronouncement. As a physician myself, I knew all too well how much sadism exists in the helping professions. Just as there is a thin line between love and hate, there is also a thin line between helping and hurting, between public safety and public endangerment. Cops and criminals, doctors and patients, lovers and haters—sometimes, it is difficult to tell the difference.

In medical training, the dividing point takes place early in the first clinical rotation during the third year of medical school. The class separates almost in half—the skittish and squeamish versus the unaffected and undaunted. The first two years of medical school are not unlike the previous sixteen years of schooling—lots of book-learning, studying, and more studying. Even the limited clinical training, the non-book learning, in the first two years of medical school is rather benign, concentrating on learning how to listen to heart sounds and lung sounds, how to look at blood vessels in the eyes, and most importantly, how to interview people and get a history of their current problems. But this all changes with the onset of rotations in pediatrics, internal medicine, surgery, and obstetrics and gynecology. Suddenly we are asked to poke and prod, stick and stab our patients whether they are infants or octogenarians.

By the second day of whatever clinical rotation we have been assigned to, we can see the impact of that first day of orientation. Half the class strides confidently off the elevator, unable to contain their enthusiasm for the opportunity to poke and prod. The other half leaves the elevator cautiously, wondering what the hell they've gotten themselves into. Somehow they—or I should say we, since I was one of this group—thought we were going to be helping people.

Instead, we were using fellow human beings as experimental fodder, stabbing them with needles ten or twenty times in order to take blood or insert IVs.

As students we could easily pick out the supersadists, the ones who immediately volunteered to do the lumbar punctures and any other invasive procedures. The spinal tap requires that you insert a needle the size of an ice pick into someone's back. A slight change in context and for that same act you're sitting in a courtroom facing a sentence of at least three to five years. Tubes put into people's urethras, cold hard speculums up vaginas, sigmoidoscopes up rectums into descending colons. In the early 1970s, before the advent of flexible fiber-optic instruments, we had only rigid instruments, all the better to inflict pain and discomfort.

Soon enough we lost track of our humanity. Even those of us who had started out skittish and squeamish became detached from the impact of what we were doing.

Is this what had happened to the urologist in New York City who was matter-of-factly sentencing me to castration? "Come up to New York City, and we'll cut off your balls." Was this a playground threat or trash-talking or bluster from a Mafia hit man?

I told myself there had to be another way to contain and control metastatic prostate cancer.

CHAPTER 1

A Death in the Family

"I would like to apologize to my family, friends, and to society as a whole for the role my penis plays in this book. I understand that no one wants to read about my sex life, but as diligently as I tried to leave him out of it, the Kid stayed in the picture."
—Nathan Rabin, *The Big Rewind*

"Baby, baby, baby, come on; what's wrong? It's a radiation vibe I'm groovin' on."
—Fountains of Wayne, "Radiation Vibe"

My pelvis died in May of 1985, after a long illness. There was no viewing since generally people who provide a viewing of their penises—whether the penis is dead or alive—are psychotic. There was no obituary since Helen and I kept the death quiet and secret—privacy for my privates. There was no funeral and burial since, well, you get the picture: How do you bury a part and not the whole?

The cause of death was not reported. But it was well-known that my pelvis had been severely mangled and maimed in prostate cancer surgery on October 5, 1984; and, just as the pelvis was in the process of recovering—urinary continence had fully returned and sexual potency was making a significant comeback—the prostate bed was hit with 6600 rads of radiation over a six-week period. Vitiated tissue no longer had the capacity to revitalize itself. The tissue had been

burned and nuked, at temperatures in the thousands of degrees—
who cared whether it was Fahrenheit or Centigrade?

The plan had been to kill every potential living cancer cell,
collateral damage be damned. The margins or borders of the tumor,
when taken out in surgery, were unclear. With the margins unclear,
the soft tissue outside of the prostate was likely to contain more than a
few prostate cancer cells. "Let's go in and nuke those motherfuckers!"
yelled the surgeons and radiation-oncologists. Except anyone who
has seen surgeons and radiation-oncologists in action knows that,
when talking to their patients, and when not behind closed doors,
they do not use that language. They are polite, soft-spoken, seemingly
thoughtful—and quite adept at quoting statistics to make their case.

In fact, the surgeons claimed they "got it all." "Don't worry,"
they were saying. "We he-men have taken care of the problem. But
just to be on the safe side, we'll have a radiation-oncologist come
talk to you about further treatment."

My pelvis hadn't quite died yet, but it was on life-support. Their
bravado was in full gear, and my swagger was more than flagging.

"You have a 40 percent chance of living up to five years and a
15 percent chance of living up to ten years," noted the radiation-
oncologist, without a bit of irony or compassion, when I engaged him
in doctor-talk. I was both a patient and a fellow doctor, but this guy
had forgotten that I was primarily the former. And I likewise had
wanted to forget that I was patient. The required role-induction in
becoming a physician had worked wonders on me. The long hours of
clinical clerkships in the last two years of medical school, the on-call
rotations of every third or every other night of my year-long internal
medicine internship had put me in a trancelike state that had allowed
me, for better or worse, to be open to a new identity. Not unlike the
marathon group therapy of Werner Erhard and EST (Erhard Seminar
Trainings) popular in the 1970s, the medical training with its sleep
deprivation and pressures not to go take a piss even when about to
pee in one's pants—lives had to be saved, diagnoses had to be made,

treatments had to be initiated—created a single-minded focus on one's identity as a physician.

—⁂—

Like so many other clinicians who had forgotten that they were husbands and wives and fathers and mothers and sons and daughters—that their identity was more than just being a doctor and caregiver—I was denying that I was a patient, a patient who was in a heap-full of trouble. Instead I was engaging in the natural one-up-man-ship of quoting survival statistics with a radiation-oncologist who, yes, knew the latest *New England Journal of Medicine* abstractions and predictions, yet who literally and concretely held my life and my morale in his hands.

So, a 40 percent chance of seeing my daughters reach the age of eleven and nine, a 15 percent chance of seeing my daughters reach their mid-teenage years. Who would want to face those odds?

If I had had any questions about what enthralled this radiation-oncologist, I found out the next day. "I got it slightly wrong," pointed out the stats nerd who must have checked the medical literature intensely the night before—better to be able to engage with his fellow doctor who was in denial about his current predicament. "You actually have a 48 percent chance of living five years, not a 40 percent chance. But I got it right about your ten-year survival. It's still 15 percent."

I could feel myself sinking deeper and deeper into the hospital bed. Just bury me now. Why wait? What happened to the dictum of Samuel Taylor Coleridge who was not only a poet but a surgeon (when surgeons were essentially barbers with scalpels), "Above all, give hope!"

Like a child without a parent or nurturer, I had to figure out how to comfort myself under the circumstances. Surgeons were good with the scalpel, radiation-oncologists were good with the rads and the data—bless them all—but few of them were comforters and nurturers. Was there any question why many people had begun to turn to alternative medical care in the latter part of the twentieth century? It was not just the hope of a new and possibly painless cure; it was also the wish to be cared for with a capital C—a capital C of caring for what was then called the big C, or cancer.

I had to give up the role induction, my identity as a physician, with all its contortions. I had to see myself in a purely "anecdotal" way. My fellow physicians generally were dismissive of any "anecdotal evidence"—evidence provided by one or two cases that might have been anomalies. Instead they preferred evidence based on a large enough sample to be able to call the findings "statistically significant"— evidence that could be used to make appropriate generalizations about the best course of action for the population at large.

Fair enough, but for my own survival I needed to discard the statistics. My own personal anecdote was paramount, not the statistics of thousands of others with the same disease.

A new spin: If my ten-year survival rate was only 15 percent, I wanted to figure out how I can be one—again, one, not hundreds— of those 15 percent. An anecdote with a good outcome, not just a statistic.

Did any of the survivors do anything special, or try any unusual treatment to enhance their chances of survival? Was it plain dumb luck, or was it just the lethal nature of the tumor that determined their chances? How much of these survival rates were within the survivors' control? Were there any commonalities among the survivors, in their treatments, their attitudes, their approaches to the cancer?

Is the past a prelude to the future? The past may be the best predictor we have for the future, but it is still hopelessly limited.

Is our personal health any different from the health of the stock market or the real estate market? As John Maynard Keynes, the economist, pointed out, "One can always cook a formula to fit moderately well a limited range of *past* facts. But what does this prove? What place is left for *expectations and the state of confidence relating to the future?* What place is allowed for non-numerical factors, such as *inventions,* labor troubles, wars, earthquakes, financial crises (emphases mine)?"

The surgeons who "got it all" had given me false hope, whereas the radiation-oncologist had given me, it turns out, a false gloom. The statistics he was showering me with were numbers from twenty to thirty years ago. No one could predict the *inventions,* the new breakthroughs in medical care in the next five or ten years. Breakthroughs had been rare in the 1960s and 1970s; the statistics were relatively static, but no one could predict the statistics would stay that way.

I had to find a way to raise *my expectations and my state of confidence.* I could not allow for self-fulfilling prophecies and the disempowerment inherent in low expectations and a low state of confidence and hope. The low survival rates for my cancer reflected this disempowerment. Many patients give up, go home to die, when faced with overwhelmingly deadly data.

The doctors were not only showering me with longevity statistics, they were also quite clear that my chances of regaining my potency were virtually zero. Too many insults to the pelvis, to the prostate bed. First surgery, then radiation—my pelvis would never recover; no one in history had ever been able to recover from that level of insult.

The lowest of low blows: The rules of boxing do not allow boxers to punch their opponent below the belt. Just in case their opponent hits them below the belt, they wear an athletic cup, a hard plastic shell to protect their testicles, their family jewels, their privates. No problem if their opponent smashes them repeatedly in the head, or anywhere else in the upper body including the arms, the chest, the abdomen, and even the kidneys.

Professional boxers do not even wear headgear to protect their brains. So, when women complain that men have their brains in their penises, they are more than half-right. We men protect our family jewels more than we protect our actual brains.

In May of 1985, I lost my fucking brain. It was now a non-fucking brain. The family jewels had been stomped on—no more fertility, no more sexual fantasies, no more sense of a sexual prowess, whatever that term means.

Athletic prowess, academic prowess, interpersonal prowess: All of these prowesses are valuable, but they do not hold a candle to sexual prowess. What does it mean to be a man, an adult male, lacking in any kind of sexual prowess? *Confidence* is shattered, *expectations* are shattered. Hopes and dreams, the pipe dreams, the fantasied, if unreal, sexual conquests—gone, kaput, crushed. No sexual prowess translates into no proudness. No self-assuredness, no brashness, no resoluteness to fight to live—instead, fragility and vulnerability.

The irony, the irony. The horror, the horror. Just a few years before, I had been teaching an honors course at the University of Maryland called "The Inner Life: The Nature of Dreams and Passions." The course, an excuse for me as a psychiatrist on campus to teach a few of my favorite Philip Roth novels including *The Professor of Desire*, *Portnoy's Complaint*, and *The Breast*, with a little John Updike and Franz Kafka thrown in for good measure, had examined our inner lives and our yearnings—our longings, especially unfilled longings, which inevitably become sexualized when we reach puberty. We looked at our dreams, our nightly reflections of our uncensored yearnings, what Sigmund Freud or his translators called "wish fulfillment."

Now a few short years later, I had become a parody of the professor of desire. A man incapable of dreams or desires or passions.

The final straw came in June of 1985, as I was sitting in our family room reading a review of a new Roth novel in the Sunday *New York Times* and realized that even the act of reading—with our imaginations aroused as we fill in the unstated blanks on the page—tied in with the penis and sex for us. The playful inner life, the playful spirit, the playful conversations, filled with playful remarks and double entendres, die with the death of the pelvis. Human touch loses a part of its meaning.

My partner, my lover—Helen—no longer had to guess whether there was any hidden meaning in a simple touch, in the holding of hands, or in an inadvertent bumping into each other while cooking together in the kitchen—a bump which under other circumstances might have led to some kisses and hugs, some looks longingly into each other's eyes that would later lead to further pleasures even if we had to wait a few hours until the kids were asleep.

As I sat in my home simply reading a book review, I could not even enjoy anything smacking of sexual playfulness. My floodgates had opened. A trivial activity, reading a newspaper, finally made me aware of how profound it is to experience the death of one's pelvis.

And it is all so private, this experience, this despair, this loss. We can talk about other losses rather readily, but not so the loss of our privates.

The word most frequently associated with the bedroom: privacy. Whatever happens in the bedroom stays in the bedroom. The gods have programmed us as a species to suddenly develop a self-consciousness, a super-awareness of our privates as soon as we reach puberty. When we suddenly have a capacity to create a new offspring—to get pregnant or make someone pregnant—we get a bit skittish about this new power, these new impulses. We cover our breasts, our vaginas, our penises obsessively, carefully, maniacally.

Even children who have grown up with nudist parents—kids who are quite inured to nudity—become highly self-conscious about their privates when they reach puberty and adolescence. No more nudity for me, thank you very much, they say. A peculiar kind of rebellion: I want my clothes on, not off.

Men who are dealing with prostate cancer, men who have faced surgery and radiation and castration suddenly clam up as well. We cover up our privates even more maniacally than ever before.

A classic example is Anthony Sattilaro who in 1982 wrote, with the help of Tom Monte, one of the earliest and most inspirational stories about his personal experiences with prostate cancer, *Recalled by Life,* a book I turned to in 1984 as I faced my own traumas. Satillaro, a physician specializing in anesthesiology, had been diagnosed with metastatic prostate cancer. By the time it was first found at the age of forty-seven, the cancer had already spread widely to his bones. Told that he had barely months to live and in hopeless despair, he unexpectedly happened upon a hitchhiker who changed his life. In a wondrous turnaround, Sattilaro took the hitchhiker's advice to try a macrobiotic diet. This diet in combination with surgical castration— the conventional treatment for metastatic prostate cancer at the time—led to the complete disappearance of visible disease. Satillaro lived for twelve more years, most of those years disease-free, before dying of the cancer.

Looking for inspiration in early 1985, with my pelvis on the verge of death, I called Satillaro. His book had focused on the near-miraculous effects of eating macrobiotically; and in his second book, he had focused on specific recipes for eating macrobiotically.

How had he dealt with castration, with the end of his sex life, with the end of double entendres and sexual playfulness? I had not faced castration yet—surgery and radiation had been bad enough— but how had he figured out how to cope? His otherwise fine book had not touched on the effects of castration, its psychological and physical impact.

"Can I ask you how you've coped with castration?" I tentatively asked, after the initial pleasantries, after some talk about our common bonds as physicians and prostate cancer sufferers. Not the usual question one asks in an initial conversation, but he was clearly supportive and cordial from the outset.

"Not so well," he noted. "I've spent hours upon hours in (psychiatric) analysis trying to cope with it. This is not easy stuff."

But not a word of these struggles in his two books. Our privates stay private especially when they have been surgically removed.

We have had *The Vagina Monologues*, and we are long overdue for *The Penis Monologues*. No better place than to start here.

CHAPTER 2

Come: Going, Going, Gone

"Hey, don't knock masturbation. It's sex with someone I love."
—Woody Allen, *Annie Hall*

Like most men, I used to be a scumbag. Now I can proudly and definitively, yet sadly, say that I am no longer a scumbag.

Facing impotence after prostate surgery at the age of thirty-six is a profound blow—a blow to one's confidence, a blow to one's sense of self, a blow to the joys of orgasm, a blow to the joys of animal spirits and passions. Yet, four to five weeks after surgery, I was feeling pretty, pretty good. I was beginning to feel my first pelvic stirrings, and I was even seeing the beginnings of erections.

The nerve-sparing procedure in taking out my prostate had worked. Instead of blindly and aggressively cutting through all the nerve supply in the pelvis to frantically pull out the prostate—the nerve supply to the pelvis is enormous, second only to the brain—the surgeons had spared virtually all of the nerves on one side of it. Theoretically this sparing of nerve damage would be enough to allow me to regain potency. And theory was turning into reality.

Everything seemed to be in sync. A friend loaned us a VCR, a new piece of technology that had just been developed in the previous year or two, and Helen and I were able to watch recently released movies at home for the first time.

I could begin to move back into denial. *I am still a twenty-
something, a teenager even, not in my mid-thirties, with the large
passions and drives of adolescence and young adulthood still going
strong. Prostate cancer, prostate surgery, future radiation to the prostate
bed: A thing of the past—the surgeons got it all, they said—and not a
thing of the future.* I am watching *Fast Times at Ridgemont High* on
the VCR, and I briefly return to my youthful innocence, unclouded
by disease and death. Helen is comforting and encouraging and
passionate. My erections are coming. A grand slam, a hole in one,
a three-point shot from half court. Thank you, Helen, thank you,
surgeons. The comeback kid is coming.

Except there was no ejaculant. A grand slam, and now bam.
No come, no scum, no jism. No muss and no fuss, as Helen quickly
reminded me. Where was it? Where did it go? I hardly knew ye.

The surprise of puberty: No more dry humping. A wet sticky
mess comes, of course, with puberty. Unless we talk with our friends,
a conversation I never had as a twelve-year-old, we have to figure out
what to do with this glutinous goo. Do we masturbate into a wad of
tissues (yes)—but then what do we do with this wad? Doesn't it look
a bit strange to suddenly be willing to empty your own small pail of
garbage every day? Doesn't it look a bit peculiar to be getting a new
box of tissues for the night table every other day? Doesn't it look
weird to make periodic trips to the trash cans outside and to take
those trash cans to the front of the house twice a week for garbage
collection—a chore I was never actually asked to do? How weird is
it to suddenly be using the washing machine and dryer a couple of
times a week, to deal with sticky underwear and sheets?

I never thought to masturbate into the toilet. It was much
more comfortable in the privacy—again, the privacy and the self-
consciousness and embarrassment of early adolescence—of my
bedroom. I never thought to use that night's yet-uncooked liver or
brisket—we were big meat eaters—as a receptacle for my newfound
fertile syrup. A new kind of meat tenderizer, a newfangled gravy

enhancer. I never thought to use an apple pie either, to bring out the juices of the apples, to make the crust as moist as possible.

And just as I am letting go of my puzzlement and my embarrassment, and just as I am enjoying the pleasures of this lush and rich and fruitful mess, it's gone. I am just as puzzled as I was at twelve. Where did it go? I had just had a modest erection, I had just had sex with Helen—something I thought might never happen ever again—I had just had an orgasm. But no ejaculant, no cum. An ejaculation without ejaculant. What the hell?

I call my internist frantically. I am experiencing orgasmic joy, I tell him; but I am completely confused. No cum came. Nothing, nada. Is there something further wrong with my penis, my pelvis, my prostate-bed?

A highly experienced physician, a few years older than myself, he was as confused as I was. "I've never heard of this. None of my patients have indicated this kind of problem post-prostatectomy previously. I'll look into it."

This was November, 1984, six weeks after surgery. Men then did not talk about sexual dysfunction, orgasms, erectile dysfunction (ED). ED was not an acronym that was anywhere close to the horizon.

I called the urological surgeon in Manhattan the next day. "Of course you're not going to have any ejaculant, any secretions. Your seminal vesicles, which produce seminal fluid, have been removed along with your prostate. The spermatic cord has been cut in the process of removing your prostate; and now the sperm, whatever is left of it, empties into your bladder. It's all retrograde ejaculation, whatever minimal fluids are left."

It has all been turned upside down.

Okay, but why didn't anyone warn me about this? It's too private. Sex stays in the bedroom, not in the surgical suite, not in the doctor's office. We've saved your life. What more do you want? We'll talk to you about survival statistics, but why should we talk to you about sexual side effects? Just deal with it. Get over it.

A new coming-of-age movie or novel for the prostate cancer generation: Where are the up-to-date renderings of *Portnoy's Complaint* and *American Pie*? How does one learn the new versions of the birds and the bees—the coming-of-age and the going-of-age? Quite possibly the confusions of puberty and adolescence are not nearly as funny as the confusions that come with prostate cancer—a new kind of self-consciousness, a new kind of stumbling and blundering and floundering.

No more human stain, no more creamy mess that keeps our species ripening and evolving. I was realizing that prostate cancer and all of its treatments affect everything that makes us human, that assures survival of us as a species.

CHAPTER 3

My Head and My Doctors' Heads Up My Butt

"I had the experience . . . of sitting on an endoscopic device (electromagnetic resonance, or some such *truc*). Inside me a balloon was inflated with water; a TV screen was turned towards me and there I saw my own prostate gland, my own seminal vesicles, my own bladder, with the fluid in it resembling a little pond with a still surface. The prostate entered the picture like the top half of an egg . . . So when my father said I had my head up my ass, this was the vision that made me laugh. What would one see there?"
—Saul Bellow, *More Die of Heartbreak*

It was not a pretty picture, what the physicians felt and saw there. I was only thirty-five years old. With his fingers up my butt, my internist told me at my yearly physical exam that my prostate was unusually enlarged for someone my age. The head of urology at a local teaching hospital told me that the size of the prostate was indeed worrisome but that I was too young to have prostate cancer. "It must be something unusual, like tuberculosis or a tubercular abscess."

If it was not cancer, I said to myself, I could put off having a metal tube put up my penis and urethra. I would just watch and wait.

A little knowledge is a dangerous thing for me as a physician. The textbooks had told me in medical school that, generally, people die *with* prostate cancer, not *of* prostate cancer. A false assumption, particularly for someone in his thirties who may have an especially aggressive form of the cancer.

Oh, if only I had had the disease of Kafka and Rilke. Tuberculosis a century ago was filled with all sorts of indignities and death. Now in the developed Western world, tuberculosis is highly treatable with antibiotics, and virtually no one dies of it unless one has an immune deficiency. No untreatable wretched coughing, no horrifying gobs of blood in the sputum, no wasting away with ghastly weight loss, no leprous isolation in an arid sanitarium.

Instead, the gods had created a new source of indignity for the late twentieth century and early twenty-first century. Those sadistic and warped gods had given up on the lungs and moved further down to the penis. So, we men could now breathe easier, but we might not be able to make love, have orgasms, and reproduce.

It starts with the male pelvic exam and only gets worse. No fun, the rectal exam with a physician's fingers up one's ass, but certainly no worse, and perhaps a bit better, than the pelvic exam for women. We men at least do not have to put our legs in stirrups but simply have to assume the doggy position.

The beginning of the end for testosterone-driven male dominance: If I ever was an alpha male, that rank no longer applies. Just stay in that doggy position and take your lumps.

—⚏—

Those lumps indeed took some disturbing new forms.

I was playing tennis with a friend on one of the two public tennis courts behind our home in northwest Washington, DC. The city had been kind enough to convert two full-court basketball courts into two tennis courts and had moved the basketball courts to another part of the park sitting behind our house. I was playing badly. My backhand had betrayed me. I was spraying my backhand shots into the net and beyond the baseline, anywhere but inside the court.

After one particularly awful shot, I had enough. Like a piqued teenager, I angrily ran over to the chain-linked fence at the back of the court and hurriedly hit a backhand into the fence. Ostensibly I was just practicing my backhand, trying to get it right for the next point. But the fence was only five feet away. The ball ricocheted weirdly and swiftly and hit me in the left testicle. A tennis ball into my balls.

No big deal, I said to myself. I finished out my tennis game. The pain was intense, but I had been through this before. I was a catcher in baseball throughout my high school years; and, when stupid enough not to wear an athletic cup, I had occasionally been hit in the balls. But the bruising and pain had resolved within a few days. Not so this time.

The pain was unremitting. I began to wonder whether my enlarged, previously asymptomatic, prostate was a more serious concern than the urologist in Washington, DC had indicated. What the hell was going on?

A bit more desperate, I made my way up to a teaching hospital in upper Manhattan—still in pain several weeks after hitting the tennis ball into my testicle. Through a friend of the family, I had been given an entrée into seeing a good young urologist at this teaching hospital, who felt my prostate and did not like what he felt. No reassurances this time that it was something benign. He took charge: "You are not going anywhere. You are not leaving the grounds of this medical center without an immediate and thorough workup. Prostate cancer absolutely has to be considered and ruled out." Thanks, I truly needed that.

Sure enough, first the ultrasound showing a large misshapen tumor that looked like anything but a benign prostate enlargement. The biopsy the next day confirmed the diagnosis. The pathology slides showed a potentially aggressive cancer, with cells that were undifferentiated, cells that were primitive and unevolved, that were dividing rapidly and refusing to die, that could readily spread throughout my body and kill me.

It was now clear that the pain in my testicles was simply a referred pain from this cancerous prostate, from an excessive neural stimulation caused by a tumor in the area.

A death sentence, at the very least a death sentence for my fertility. I may, at the time, not have known about the end of my ejaculant; but I did know that now at the age of thirty-six I would indeed be infertile after surgery. Helen and I had been trying for a third child the previous year without success, a failing possibly related to the developing cancer.

"How about if I spend tonight and whatever time I have before surgery masturbating so that we can collect and save and freeze my sperm for the future," I asked the surgeon. I had begun to see spanking the monkey in biblical terms. Every last mobile sperm cell was precious and deserved an opportunity to head up the vaginal canal and duke it out with its brethren in order to inseminate one of Helen's eggs.

His response took me aback, "You are facing a lethal disease. How can you possibly be focused on an issue as frivolous as fertility when your life is hanging in the balance? This is not the time to think about having another child."

If I was not preoccupied with thoughts of death before this conversation, I was now totally obsessed. If, as W. H. Auden pointed out, "Lust is less a physical need than a way of forgetting time and death," then with lust now verboten, time and death were the only elements of life I was allowed to think about, according to this expert who had my life in his hands.

With the 20/20 vision of hindsight do I now know that reports of my impending death were greatly exaggerated. Sitting here reasonably healthy and vibrant thirty years after the radical prostatectomy, I now know that Helen and I could have had a third child, a child who might have finished college by this time, a child who might have moved on to his or her adult life, a child who might have been raised by an intact family, with a relatively intact father in the picture. If seventy-year-old men can have the hubris to father young children and assume they will live into their children's adulthood, then physicians cannot assume they can predict the longevity and survival of their patients, even ones with an apparent death sentence hanging over their heads.

Never underestimate the survival instincts of a patient. Never underestimate the possibility of medical breakthroughs in enhancing that survival. Never assume you know how lucky or unlucky a person will be in their length of days. Never tell a man or woman they cannot bring a child into the world, when that child can be a life-giving force in the face of death. Never play god with a patient. Your knowledge of the future is just as limited as anyone else's.

Never tell a man not to follow his lust, not to spank the monkey, when he is in the midst of grappling with prostate cancer.

CHAPTER 4

What Is the Prostate?

"Each ejaculation contains several billion sperm cells—
or roughly the same number as there are people in the
world—which means that, in himself, each man holds
the potential of an entire world . . . As Leibniz put it:
'Every living substance is a perpetual living mirror of the
universe.'"

—Paul Auster, *The Invention of Solitude*

"Human strength will not endure to dance without cessation;
and everyone must reach the point at length of absolute
prostration."

—Lewis Carroll

The prostate: The one unpronounceable word in medical school.
Even in the fifth edition of *Shearer's Manual of Human Dissection*, a
book I used in my first semester human anatomy class, the prostate
is listed as the "prostrate" in the index.

Later, when I was practicing internal medicine before moving
into psychiatry, I would be asked by male patients after a rectal
exam, "How's my prostrate, doc?" "Your prostrate feels fine," I would
reply, going along with their humble pronunciation, knowing I could
pronounce it no better.

The prostate is a chestnut-shaped organ at the base of the penis in the lower pelvis, partly muscular and partly glandular. It secretes a milky fluid that is discharged into the urethra at the time of the emission of semen, the discharge thus mixing with the seminal fluid from the seminal vesicles at the time of ejaculation and orgasm. The bilateral seminal vesicles lie just above the base of the prostate. The fluid from the seminal vesicles and the prostate empty into the vas deferens, filled with sperm cells from the testicles, to form the fertile ejaculant that perpetuates our species. Interestingly, the seminal vesicles are resistant to virtually all of the disease processes that affect the prostate—no inflammations (as in prostatitis), no cancers.

The word "prostate" comes from the Latin "pro" and "stata," formerly from the Greek "pro" and "statos." The prostate stands as a "guardian"—something "placed" and "standing." In other words, if one loses one's prostate, from cancer and its various treatments, one loses one's guardian. Indeed one is barely left standing; one's penis can barely stand up straight. Losing the prostate can lay a man low—well-nigh prostrate.

—⁓—

Only mammals have prostates. As female mammals developed mammary glands to feed their young, the males developed prostate glands at the same time.

Male cats and dogs have prostates; all the male apes and monkeys have prostates, as do bulls and male elephants,

Not all mammals have seminal vesicles. Carnivorous mammals—meat-eaters like lions—do not have seminal vesicles. For some peculiar reason, not having seminal vesicles while being a meat-eater protects an animal from developing prostate cancer. Almost all animals that have both prostates and seminal vesicles are herbivores—vegetable-eating animals like bulls, apes, and elephants.

Human males are the exception to the rule: We are virtually the only mammalian males who have both the prostate and seminal vesicles and who also eat meat. Our closest evolutionary relative—the pygmy chimp or bonobo—has seminal vesicles and a prostate and only eats fruits and vegetables and greens. Bonobos never develop prostate cancer.

We humans are too clever for our own good. We have planted the seeds for our own destruction—if not the destruction of our species, then at least the destruction of our prostates. When our evolutionary predecessors 600,000 years ago developed the capacity to cook, we became committed carnivores. When the earth's climate and temperatures stabilized 10,000 to 12,000 years ago, we human beings began to domesticate animals. We quit running after animals and instead began to herd them and breed them in captivity. We also became much more sedentary.

The only other animal to develop clinically significant prostate cancer with any regularity is the dog—the pet that eats from our human table, the pet that eats virtually the same food—and meat—as people.

The prostate and its ruination via prostate cancer may truly be the ultimate sentinel, the ultimate tiny chestnut-shaped canary in the human coal mine. This highly vulnerable organ is indeed trying to tell us something essential. We ignore this organ at our own risk.

CHAPTER 5

My So-Called Life

"I read where you don't suffer comforters lightly, but I have to tell you I was shocked to read about your (prostate) cancer. It doesn't pay to write a wonderful story like 'What the Cystoscope Said' not so long as Aristophanes is God."
　　—From a letter from Philip Roth to Anatole Broyard

"God is the greatest comedian but He's playing to an audience too afraid to laugh."
　　　　　　　　　　　　　　　　　　　　　—Voltaire

No comedy within miles. All tragedy. It was the day after my experience of reading the Philip Roth review in the *New York Times* in May of 1985. It was the end of the academic year at the University of Maryland where I had been a staff psychiatrist at the University Health Center for the past four and a half years. It was now two months post-radiation and seven months post-surgery. All I had was dead pelvis on the mind.

I was leading a psychotherapy group, the final one of the semester before the summer break. A couple of students were graduating; a couple of others were finishing up a year or two of treatment and were ready to move on with their lives without therapy. Several others would continue in the group in the coming academic year. We were all saying our good-byes.

The group already knew from previous leavings that we had a ritual for these departures. We gave the parting member a psychological gift, and the parting member returned the favor: We shared with that member our appreciations and resentments, our hopes and fears for this patient. We recognized the psychological and emotional accomplishments of this patient in his or her therapy; and we acknowledged the potential psychological pitfalls this patient may face in the future, given his or her specific emotional vulnerabilities. The departing member shared his or her appreciations and resentments about the others in the group, including me.

What a boon, what a reward for all of us. Even in a group that had as its most significant value that of openness and honesty, we could be more open and honest when we are exiting, when we had less fears of inadvertently hurting someone. Just as parents learn the most about parenting from their children, I as a psychiatrist learn the most from my patients—how I could have handled situations differently, what helped and what did not help, what they may have resented about my interactions with them.

Group therapy can be remarkably powerful with young adults, with undergraduates and graduate students. There is no better way to break through shame and self-consciousness, no better way to create an environment of unconditional acceptance, an experience that may never have occurred during some members' childhoods. There is no better way to recognize that one is not alone, that others are experiencing similar struggles, that others are experiencing seemingly worse problems than one's own. There is no better way to begin to trust one's own instincts and beliefs, to recognize one's own therapeutic capabilities, in helping others as well as oneself, without necessarily having to rely on the therapist, the so-called authority. Students begin to develop their own voice, to recognize their own authority. This evolution of their own voice culminates in their sharing with me and the rest of the group their appreciations and resentments as they leave the group. When a group clicks, it becomes a corrective emotional experience for everyone in the group—and a deeply gratifying experience for me as a psychiatrist.

Not so that day. A brain fog, a blur. *Dead pelvis . . . Dead penis . . . Dead pelvis.* For the first time in my professional career, I was simply going through the motions. I was unable to compartmentalize, unable to keep my personal problems separate from my work.

One of the students, a Trinidadian woman who had been in the group for over two years, approached me after the ninety-minute session. "Dr. Steinberg, did you forget that I am graduating next week?" she asked quietly and sheepishly and forlornly.

"Oh, my goodness. What was I thinking? Of course I knew you were graduating. I am so, so sorry. I cannot believe that we forgot to share with you our hopes and fears for you and we forgot to hear your feedback. I don't know what happened to my brain today." I knew all too well what happened to my brain, to my whole body. I stood there cringing. I could barely stop from cursing at myself.

She did not have to remind me that graduating from the University of Maryland was no small deal to her. She was the first in her family to ever have gone to college and to seek out psychiatric help and to overcome the stigma of psychiatry in her culture. Whatever problems and struggles her family may have had, she was not going to pass it on to the next generation.

She did not have to remind me how seriously I took my work. In the seven years since completing my psychiatry residency, I had come to recognize the profound and almost blind trust that patients place in me—me, a person who was a perfect stranger until that first meeting with them. To hear a student's emotional distress, to know that he or she has reached the end of his or her tether: It filled me with awe that people had enough faith and confidence in me and my professional abilities to open up about the most shattering and shameful parts of their lives. A public trust that I had never wanted to betray.

I had forgotten to give this young woman a final gift from me and the group. She had not had the opportunity to give her final gift to the group. No closure. The group, for her, had died with barely a whimper.

Despite the diminishing stigma about mental health care in the past twenty-five years, this was still 1985. No one came to a psychiatrist without some trepidation and hesitation. My public trust was to make that experience as comfortable and pleasant and rewarding and beneficial as possible. Abiding by the Hippocratic Oath—"Above all, do no harm"—was not nearly enough. For college students, it was essential that they had a truly constructive and valuable experience. Their lives were very much ahead of them, and it was crucial for them to feel comfortable seeking out further treatment, if necessary, in the future.

Months later, with some bitterness, she let me know that I "must not have cared enough" about her to recognize the milestone of her graduation and the significance of her leaving therapy.

It was one thing for my despair, my dead pelvis, my distractions, to affect me and only me; it was quite another for this despair to have a profound effect on my patients, on Helen, on my daughters. The despair did not come right away, when the pelvis died. No, it came weeks later with the events of everyday life—a simple article in a book review section, a devastating mistake in my day-to-day professional routine. Then I asked, as did Tolstoy's Ivan Ilyich, "What is this for? . . .Why all this horror? What is it for?"

"You're a good candidate for a penile implant," noted my surgeon, not surprised at all by my impotence and dead pelvis. Yeah, just what I need—a piece of plastic with a balloon apparatus stuffed into my penis. Leave my fucking (or non-fucking) penis alone, I wanted to shout into the phone. "I'll think about it," I politely replied.

"Boxers box," said A. J. Liebling. And surgeons? Wind them up and they only do surgery. I needed something different for now. No more surgical interventions. Let everything heal to whatever extent it can from the prostatectomy and the radiation. Let me ponder my predicament for a bit.

Can I use this horror, this despair, this muddle as a call to action? I wanted to do something. But what? My helplessness, and the powerlessness of my physicians, was palpable. My so-called life was a mess.

CHAPTER 6

Mesmerized

"Nothing that befalls anyone is ever too senseless to have happened."

—Philip Roth

"When a man knows he is to be hanged in a fortnight, it concentrates his mind wonderfully."

—Samuel Johnson

It was all so retro. In the midst of my confusion and despair and helplessness in the months after surgery and radiation, I turned to the nineteenth century, to Franz Anton Mesmer and to Ivan Pavlov for guidance and mentorship. Unlike Pavlov, however, I was looking for salvation, not salivation.

Mesmer was the Google of the eighteenth century, the first name or noun that became a verb. Just as we might google now, people in eighteenth century Europe became mesmerized. Hypnosis, or mesmerism, played a significant role in the peculiar history of psychiatry, with Mesmer having been one of the earliest influences on Sigmund Freud. In 1779 in his dissertation "Mesmerism: The Discovery of Animal Magnetism," Mesmer hypothesized that human beings were endowed with a special magnetic fluid, a kind of sixth sense, which when liberated could produce near-miraculous healing effects. Until controversy and charges of quackery curtailed his career, Mesmer claimed to have magnetized and cured hundreds of patients, many of whom would be considered now to have had what we call psychological conversion reactions, such as hysterical blindness and hysterical paralyses.

Had Mesmer helped to heal people with cancers or other deadly illnesses, diseases that now can be defined and delineated by pathology slides and X-rays? No one knows, but several of his disciples were able to use hypnosis or mesmerism as a method of anesthetizing and treating patients in India and England. Had Mesmer been able to see something, this magnetic fluid, that none of the rest of us had been able to see? No one knows.

In his epilogue to *War and Peace*, Leo Tolstoy, fascinated with hypnosis, wondered what allowed certain armies to win battles and wars and what allowed various peoples to make major migrations, from west to east or east to west, or, in apocryphal biblical terms, from inside Egypt to an exodus outside of Egypt. Some kind of powerful force might be able to drive us to unimaginable heights. We have all seen it—a force that allows an athletic team to be beautifully synchronized so that the whole is greater than the sum of its parts, and the team achieves more than anyone could have expected.

All I had been looking for was some semblance of control. Helpless, helpless, helpless. Was it possible for me, though, to synchronize all of my efforts, to pull together all of my powers, to have access to my magnetic fluids or sixth sense in order to stay alive as long as possible? To alter the quality of my life in such a way as to regain some semblance of being a sexual being? Could I find a way to create good team chemistry within my body—for all my organs and tissues and cells to be working in a coordinated way—in an effort to live a rich and full life? No self-sabotage allowed. No Freudian death instinct allowed. No self-destruction allowed.

—m—

The day before I left the hospital in Manhattan in mid-October of 1984, after the prostatectomy, I called an old medical colleague of mine who was versed in the Simonton approach to cancer treatment. Designing a program to maximize one's sense of control in the face of abject powerlessness, Carl Simonton, a radiation-oncologist, and his wife Stephanie Matthew-Simonton, a psychotherapist, developed an approach that used mental imagery to help in recovery. Their premise, bizarre in retrospect, was that the cancer patient had caused his own demise and thus had the power to undo his own demise. Yes, blame oneself and blame the victim. The fault is not in the stars but in ourselves.

The Simontons described cancer patients who believed they had somehow "made" themselves ill. Forget about the possibility of simply being star-crossed. We somehow can believe we have complete control over our destiny.

Exactly what I needed at the time. Desperate circumstances require desperate measures. With the help of the Simontons, I now deluded myself into thinking it was not only radiation that was killing any remaining cancer cells; it was also my mental imagery.

The imagery? My medical colleague has asked me to draw an image of my immune system cells as well as an image of the cancer cells. Hardly an artist, I took out some colored pencils at home and came up with an image of a vivid Venus flytrap-like plant with enormous magenta flowers plucking tiny black and yellow bugs from the air. Plucking insects and destroying them—a primitive set of Pac-Men as killer T-cells trapping and swallowing any now-fragile and vulnerable irradiated cancer cells. Hardly the most aggressive image, I saw these plants as a lean, mean fighting machine swallowing up those all-too-deadly cancer cells.

I convinced myself: My mind and body were working in a fully synchronized way with the cancer treatments. I was not a passive victim and observer. Instead I was an active participant in the eradication of cancer cells.

How nutty but necessary.

Cancer patients in 1984 had to run the gauntlet of psychological theories about cancer. The most prominent theory was that cancer patients were not able to express anger and other emotions effectively. A blocked-up psyche, they claimed. Let's add insult to injury. But I had no trouble with blocked-up anger and repressed emotions. These theories simply made me furious. Energized, I was ready to take on cancer and the theorists.

Susan Sontag was on my side in recognizing the over-psychologizing of illness. Historically, as Susan Sontag pointed out in *Illness as Metaphor*, the amount of psychological theorizing about a particular illness is directly proportional to the mysteriousness of the disease, to how little is known of its cause. Up until the late nineteenth century, virtually nothing was known about the causes of tuberculosis. Koch's postulates, recognizing the significance of microorganisms as causative agents for diseases like tuberculosis, had not been put forth yet. So, psychological theories about the causes of tuberculosis abounded.

These theories died a welcome death as soon as the tubercle bacillus was discovered. With cancer, these psychological theories have only recently begun to recede as we learn more about viruses and toxic chemicals and radiation and cell aging and immune system deficiencies as causes for the disease.

Yet, when our lives are out of our control, when we find ourselves in a grim situation for no clear-cut reason, we will go to extraordinary lengths to find some cockamamie approach to re-establish some semblance of control. Then, when we find the root of our predicament, we assume we can find an antidote, a solution. If we do not find it, we have only ourselves to blame—for causing the illness and not being able to cure it. What Joshua Cody calls "the guilt of the ill."

The Simontons, however, allowed me to feel that I could actively do something, anything, to augment the effects of the actual medical treatments. And, more importantly, the Simontons inadvertently reintroduced me to the work of Ivan Pavlov.

Pavlov was the progenitor of the notion of the anchoring stimulus, a ubiquitous phenomenon that we are only beginning to understand and appreciate. In his simple but exquisitely elegant experiments, Pavlov put powdered meat in front of hungry dogs and watched as their entire digestive physiology changed. These dogs began to salivate, and the chemistry of their stomachs and intestines began to change as well. If Pavlov rang a bell at the same time that he put powdered meat in front of these starving dogs, the bell then became an anchoring stimulus. And if Pavlov repeated this protocol for five successive days—ringing a bell at the same time meat was offered—the bell alone, even without food, became the only stimulus needed to create the physiological changes in the dogs' guts. Salivation and chemical changes in the gut, just with the ringing of a bell.

Pavlov used other stimuli besides a bell, including whistles, tuning forks, and metronomes, as well as visual stimuli, all of which are now considered anchoring stimuli in the psychological world of conditioned responses.

Anchoring stimuli and conditioned responses are everywhere. They create the reflex reaction in post-traumatic stress. If we are in a war zone and hear explosions repeatedly, all it takes is a loud noise to change our entire physiology, to trigger the startle response, a huge adrenaline rush, and an all-consuming fear.

Mild traumas occur virtually every day of our lives. Conditioned responses get triggered virtually every day of our lives. Physiological reactions—in our central nervous system and in our gut—get triggered virtually every day of our lives.

Is there some way to bottle these reactions in a benign way? Again, I wanted redemption and salvation, not salivation. I wanted to harness my immune system, change its physiology, and bolster its responses to a threat from within.

I followed up with a hypnotherapist whom my medical colleague referred me to. He urged me to take the images to another level—to wear clothes that were pink or purple or magenta—because he believed they were visual anchoring stimuli that could possibly change my physiology and power my immune system.

I ended up making these colors ubiquitous—pants, shirts, sweaters, socks, underwear, watches, caps, jackets, you name it. Even cordovan loafers. I also began to meditate for five minutes every hour (thank the gods for the forty-five to fifty-minute hour in psychiatric practice). I was constantly focused on my recovery, consciously when meditating and unconsciously when inadvertently looking at my watch or socks. Those killer Venus flytrap T-cells were in my head for every waking hour.

With my knowledge of Pavlovian reflexes, I recognized how much I wanted some kind of immediate automatic reminder, conscious and unconscious, of my cancer and my killer T-cells; and I knew that I was going to need pink and magenta, coincidentally my two daughters' favorite colors, to become an everyday part of my life. Every upcoming day of my life, I realized, I would be wearing pink and purple shirts and socks, that despite the lack of proof of its value I would somehow keep the faith in these hues and would give up earth colors, every brown and every yellow and every green, forever.

—w—

My purple phase: Jimi Hendrix's "Purple Haze" and Prince's "Purple Rain" and Tommy James's "Crimson and Clover" became my anthems. I made sure Alice Walker's *The Color Purple* was prominently displayed on my bookshelf.

Given my daughters' favorite colors, I asked for their assistance in making over my wardrobe.

Then I came across a book by Bernie Siegel, a cancer surgeon in Connecticut. In *Love, Medicine, and Miracles* he expresses his belief that images of immune cells conceived in a purplish spectrum—as opposed to a black or yellow hue—will give them greater power and strength. Who was I to argue?

I took my effort at salvation to an even higher level. Just before I started radiation therapy to my prostate bed in January 1985, three months after prostate surgery, I went up to New York City by myself to listen to a young man in his mid-twenties convince a group of two hundred people to walk across twenty feet of burning, steaming charcoals within the following two hours after he had trained us how to do so.

He and his assistants set up two rows of gray and red burning charcoals—charcoals on which any of us could cook steaks and hamburgers—to test our flesh and our willingness to challenge conventional wisdom, to defy assumptions about what is doable and not doable. The coals were sitting on a small messy grass lawn outside a crumbling hotel overlooking thirty-fourth Street and Penn Station and Madison Square Garden. Again, early 1985: The city itself was a shell of its former grandeur, with weed-filled grassy areas waiting for office towers to be built. But it was a perfect and desolate place for a barbecue pit for human flesh, human soles.

In 1985 it was uncertain whether New York City would make a comeback, and even more uncertain whether I would make a comeback. My pelvis was facing the same kind of desolation as Manhattan.

Tony Robbins was our guide for this evening. An unknown at the time, he later turned his fire walking and inspirational exhortations into a television career and occasional film appearances. His events later attracted up to six thousand people at a time; and these fire-walking experiences were featured and skewered in films like *Down and Out in Beverly Hills*. I was merely one of the early initiates.

I had a specific agenda, though—a quite concrete and literal agenda—to survive the burning of my pelvis. If I could walk across blazing hot coals and not develop first or second or third degree burns, I told myself, then I may be able to survive the enormous heat from radiation to the pelvis. For me this was no spiritual walk with symbolic significances. I was not looking at larger existential questions. No efforts to figure out the boundaries of human capabilities—no nonsense about the triumph of the human spirit. This was just pure firefighting. "Save my soles," not "Save my soul."

I was fighting fire . . . with not exactly fire. And Mesmer and Pavlov, all embodied in Tony Robbins's expertise, were my comrades fighting the upcoming pelvic fire.

A magnetic and mesmerizing, yet approachable, figure, Robbins got the crowd into a highly relaxed and focused and suggestible state. He repeatedly reminded us that he had led these hot coal walks hundreds of times with nary an injury. "Calm confidence" was a mantra he instilled in us—a confidence in ourselves and a confidence we began to have in him.

Not surprisingly, he used a specific anchoring stimulus. "As you begin to feel calmer and safer and more confident, raise your left arm as high as you can and then bring your right hand up to meet the left hand. As this feeling of calmness and confidence takes hold, make a fist with your right hand."

Adolph Hitler had nothing on us. In the midst of this surreal scene in midtown Manhattan, I could see the remarkable power of a Hitler, someone who, as unschooled as he might have been, harnessed the power of an anchoring stimulus. He was able to get his audience into a super aroused state and then anchor that state by associating it with the heil-Hitler Nazi salute, a salute so elegant in its simplicity. He was able to put an entire country into an almost irresistible trance, a trance he then used to instill an exaggerated view of the German Aryan people as a people and as warriors—views that were not at all at odds with how they wished to view themselves.

Robbins used some simple suggestions to allow us to walk calmly and confidently across the molten coals. "Walk purposefully and assuredly, and not too quickly, across the coals. Do not run." Apparently tripping on hot coals is not a good idea.

He invoked an image of "cool moss." We were to repeatedly utter "cool moss" out loud as we walked over the coals, as this was another anchoring stimulus to go along with the tightened right fist—an effort to have us believe something that was diametrically opposite to the image emanating from the molten coals themselves. And indeed, as I recited "cool moss," my physiology changed dramatically. I began to look forward to the walk, to the cool moss under my feet, instead of dreading it.

Mind over matter. There is something to it, I thought. I *will* make it across these coals safely. And after radiation I will go forth purposefully and assuredly, not in a hasty and desperate way. Cool moss in the pelvis as well.

I made it across the coals without incident. A few blisters popped up on the bottom of my feet but were gone within twenty-four hours. Less complications than after exposure to the midday Mediterranean summer sun.

—⁓—

We all are at our maximal hypnotizable state, or level of suggestibility, by age nine. This hypnotizability increases gradually from birth until it peaks at nine, then begins to slowly tail off until we lose most of our suggestibility by age nineteen or twenty. From an evolutionary standpoint, this trajectory makes perfect sense: We come into this world as a blank slate, needing older and wiser authority figures, usually our parents, our teachers, our older siblings, to show us the ropes. Our heightened suggestibility allows us to be open to these mentors and advisors, even if they might lead us astray or even brainwash us.

By the age of twenty, we no longer need this suggestibility. We can think on our own, we can even develop a bit of skepticism and cynicism, a worldliness that allows us to make our own decisions about the paths we may follow.

In facing a death sentence, and at the very least the death of my pelvis, I was counting on returning to a childlike state of suggestibility that would allow me to be more open to any authority figures who might have some answers and antidotes. I could only hope to find the right masters who would not lead me astray.

I came to realize that the power of hypnosis was not with the hypnotic trance itself but with the suggestions connected with the trance. The trance is simply a heightened state of relaxation, concentration, and focus. The trance is simply the vehicle or substrate through which we can fully absorb an idea or suggestion. The suggestion is the thing.

"Cool moss," "Walk purposefully and assuredly, and not too quickly," were crucial suggestions for making it across twenty feet of steaming coals without major burns. What kind of hypnotic suggestion could I turn to in making it through the ravages of surgery and radiation as well as the prostate cancer itself?

One of the best hypnotherapists at coming up with the most optimal suggestions was Milton Erikson. Practicing in the shadows of Las Vegas, he was able to intervene effectively and quickly with gambling problems, sexual dysfunctions, and tobacco addictions, all the problems endemic to Las Vegas. Single session treatments—one and done. His childhood affliction with polio—and his extended, though not permanent, paralysis at a tender age—forced him to be an observer, less a participant, in his early life. He was able to recognize the nuances of facial expressions and body postures, offhanded comments, and subtle resistances as family members and neighbors interacted with each other—nuances that the rest of us do not pick up on in our more active childhoods. His astuteness allowed him to take the measure of the people whom he was treating and to come up with the shrewdest of suggestions for use during the hypnotic trance, suggestions that were clever and perfectly designed.

With the astuteness and wisdom of a Milton Erikson, my hypnotherapist came up with what turned out to be a life-altering hypnotic suggestion. As I entered a deepening state of relaxation, with guided imagery conveying me to ladders and stairs that brought me deeper and deeper into the rich root system of a tree and on into a wondrous tapestry of vivid colors and sounds and smells and tastes, he suggested that I focus on the following thought:

> *I will do everything I can, everything humanly possible, not only to survive the prostate cancer but also to bring my sexual life back to full health. I will go to the ends of the earth if necessary to find medical interventions that can allow me to have a full return of sexual capacities and to preserve my life.*

This hypnotic suggestion became my mantra, my vow. No actions to be taken now, but there might be plenty of action to take after the dust from radiation and surgery settled.

So, for five to ten minutes every hour, I focused on relaxing and putting myself into a trance, guiding myself into a state in which I could engrain the thought, "I will do everything I can to save my life and bring my pelvis back to life."

Yes, I was in a trance for five minutes every hour. I was focusing on images of Venus flytrap-like plants swallowing up any random cancer cells for five minutes every hour. I was wearing purple and pink clothes that kept me vigilant about cancer for every waking minute. But this trance did not seem to be impeding my work, my family life, or my social life. If anything, these vows and mantras and trances allowed me to function pretty damn well.

Every one of us is in some kind of trance every day. We only recognize this when we find ourselves, say, at EXIT 8 of the New Jersey Turnpike after seemingly just having passed EXIT 2. Driving for us has become effortless, automatic. But nothing we learn is initially automatic. It is effortful, requiring the slow and deliberate thinking that Daniel Kahneman, the psychologist and Nobel prizewinner in economics, has described. So it is with hypnosis and the trance and the suggestions and vows and mantras. Effortful, and gradually becoming effortless—the fast thinking and automatic thinking that come with doing something over and over and over again.

We have work trances—especially when we have been in a job for months and years. We have personal life trances—especially when our personal lives have developed a certain routine. We have family gathering trances—especially when we have dealt with our families repeatedly over the years. We put ourselves into a slightly different mode depending on the venue and audience, and we integrate all of these different modes and trances and effortless capabilities into one genuine whole.

I am simply adding an additional mode, or channel, to my television box, a new channel that is turned on twenty-four hours each day, providing background noise most of the time and then coming into the foreground for five to ten minutes every hour. This channel—and these trances—is no longer random and inadvertent. Instead, they are a highly purposeful part of my life. The trance allows me to relax, to remove myself from the stress of day-to-day life. The vow allows me to face the future, not give up, have some sense of control, and gain confidence that my life can take a turn for the better.

Cool moss in the face of hot coals, the ends of the earth for interventions in the face of prostate cancer and the ravages of its treatment.

—⁓—

As a psychiatrist I often see the impact of powerful vows taken in childhood—vows taken between, say, the ages of eight and ten that have both positive and negative consequences in adulthood. Examples: A sensitive child who has grown up with a violent and abusive parent, vowing that he will be the antithesis of that parent in his behavior as an adult. A child who is a witness to a hateful and vicious marriage of her parents, vowing, if not a life of chastity, at least an avoidance of permanent relationships. Likewise a child who has watched an older sibling destroy his parents and family with rebellion and drug problems, vowing total compliance, unmitigated obedience—never wanting to rock the boat as an adult, never wishing to take risks that might lead to distress in friends and partners, and thus forsaking a fuller and richer life.

Freud may have been mistaken in his belief that the "latency period" between the ages of five and puberty is merely a time of consolidation and a regrouping after the novel stimulations of the first five years of life and before the hormonal turmoil of adolescence. Instead, during this period of heightened suggestibility and hypnotizability, this so-called latency is hardly a period of dormancy. We are establishing a set of beliefs, a modus operandi, which is virtually impossible to shake in adulthood, except with considerable therapeutic effort.

The perfect example of vow power: The comedian Stephen Colbert has talked of the impact of a remarkable vow he made at the age of ten. His father and two older brothers had just died in a horrific plane crash in Charlotte, North Carolina. Leaving the funeral in a limousine with two older sisters—Colbert is the youngest of eleven children—Colbert watched in amazement as one of his sisters told a joke or said something hilarious that made the other sister roll on the floor of the limousine with uncontrolled laughter. Colbert made a vow that he appears to be keeping for the rest of his life. Here is my version of it:

> *I will do everything I can to make people laugh—to laugh in the face of adversity, to laugh in the face of tragedy. I want to be able to make people laugh in the way that my sister made my other sister laugh uncontrollably, to make people roll on the floor, to forget their immediate troubles even in the face of destruction and distress and death. I will make a career out of making people live and die laughing.*

Hilarity in the face of helplessness, a temporary denial of death in the face of undeniable distress. An openness, a suggestibility we have at the age of nine or ten—an openness, a suggestibility we have in the face of our feeling the most fragile and vulnerable.

In the face of my helplessness and defenselessness, I realized that whatever vow I took would be with me for the rest of my life, whether that life lasted less than five years or more than twenty-five years. This vow was to be constructive and nourishing and restorative. I could not afford a vow that limited the fullness and richness of life. I wanted this vow possibly to extend my life but also to make that life very much worth living.

The vow I took had several advantages. It reflected what I call a "growth mind-set," to use a term coined by Carol Dweck at Stanford University. I was not committing myself to a fixed and rigid outcome, nor was I falsely reassuring myself of a happy ending and positive results. All I committed to was the *effort* to go to all ends of the earth to achieve the kind of outcome I wanted. No guarantees. I may die relatively soon; I might die a thousand small deaths with the death of my pelvis.

My vow was also grounded in reality, the reality of death and destruction. As valuable as a denial of death can be, this denial also insulates us from an abject terror that can be a monumental positive motivating force.

My vow did not have a base of false optimism. Yes, it was grounded in the typical can-do perspective of us Americans. But it was a can-do of going to the ends of the earth, not a can-do of "I will cure myself of this disease, I will win this battle, and I will undoubtedly heal my pelvis." I was filled with doubts and terrors, all pushing me to follow that vow to go anywhere and everywhere to preserve my life and regain some semblance of sexual health. The overwhelming obstacles I was facing could also be opportunities.

It was impossible to know where my vow might lead. The regeneration of the salamander's tail was just in its nascent stages.

CHAPTER 7

The Salamander: Can We Humans Regenerate?

"God gave men both a penis and a brain, but unfortunately not enough blood supply to run both at the same time."
—Robin Williams

The salamander is my, and perhaps everyone's, model and inspiration for regeneration. Salamanders have a capacity to regenerate their tails, legs, retinas, even their spinal cords and parts of internal organs like the heart, whenever these body parts are lost or partially destroyed.

For a species to have a regenerative capacity, it must have an appendage that is not absolutely essential—one that can be lost for a period of time while regeneration occurs. Yet this appendage must be important enough that its regeneration provides a selective advantage by evolutionary standards.

My penis fits the bill.

The penis is not absolutely essential for survival. It can go about its business wounded for a while without one's life being in mortal danger. But its regeneration offers a clear-cut selective advantage for any man fighting to thrive, not just survive, in an alpha-male dominated world.

We humans, not unlike salamanders, can develop primitive dedifferentiated cells in response to injury, cells that are actually stem cells. In salamanders these cells can later evolve and differentiate into cells that are specific to a certain organ or body part. Our human cells, however, do not have this capacity to differentiate; they instead can become proliferating cancer cells, unwilling and unable to die according to the precepts of a programmed cell death. They keep on living—nothing can stop them from proliferating. Injuries caused by, say, radiation or ultraviolet rays or viruses can lead to this creation of primitive dedifferentiated stem cells that turn into cancers.

In contrast, the salamander's dedifferentiated cells are able to transform themselves, to migrate to the place in which they are supposed to function, to develop into cells that create muscle, nerve fibers, connective tissue, and blood vessels in a leg or a tail or a retina. These evolving cells allow the salamander to return to its normal functioning as a whole being.

These primitive vertebrates are able to generate an enormous electrical current at the wound site. This current in turn creates voltage gradients that allow the gradually differentiating cells to sense their position and to grow outward, to grow in the appropriate direction to regenerate the limb that has been lost.

Salamanders do not appear to develop cancers. You can inject them with the most carcinogenic drug imaginable, and still no cancer comes into play. Maybe at most an ectopic or extra limb, but no cancer.

More highly developed vertebrates like ourselves have lost the capacity to regenerate limbs and organs. In evolving into warm-blooded animals, we have needed the capability to develop scar tissue over wounds as rapidly as possible. Pathogens, including bacteria, thrive and proliferate in warm temperatures, in the warm blood of warm-blooded animals. We need to seal off wounds quickly.

Cold-blooded species can survive for months without eating, whereas birds and mammals would starve to death. And, if birds and mammals were to be crippled for any length of time during regeneration of a leg or retina, they would become easy prey. Not so the salamander.

Salamanders can sit under a log for weeks without eating or doing anything while their body part regenerates. All the salamander needs is some modicum of nerve supply to the injured organ and some electrical current between the outside of the body and the inside—just ten to one hundred millivolts or microamperes per square centimeter. And voila: as long as skin and scar tissue—the salamander is incapable of producing scar tissue—do not block the electrical current and the healing process, a brand-new organ or limb soon reappears.

—⁊⁊—

The humiliations and indignities of prostate cancer and the wounds in my pelvis and the enormous amount of scar tissue ultimately were pushing me to focus on the possibilities of some kind of regeneration. But, despite our best efforts, we human beings cannot replicate the regeneration process of salamanders. We are limited by our humanness; we are limited by our warm-bloodedness. And at the same time we are enlarged by our humanness, by our warm-bloodedness. With warm-bloodedness comes the evolution of the human brain, arguably the most remarkable evolutionary development—the most remarkable organ—in the history of our planet.

So, we go from cold-bloodedness to braininess; we go from regeneration of limbs and organs to scar tissue and cancers. All we can do is take what evolution gives us. We lose some remarkable capabilities while we gain even more remarkable capabilities.

Here's the thing: The brain and the pelvis are highly intertwined. The pelvic region is second only to the brain in the amount of neural tissue it contains. This pelvic neural tissue, along with the associated neurohormones—testosterone and estrogen and progesterone and oxytocin, to name a few—stimulate our desire to reproduce . . . to create with each successive generation our constantly evolving brains.

In my efforts to re-establish life in my penis, I may have altered the synapses in my cerebral cortex. A rebooting, a new kind of regeneration, a new kind of cerebral evolution, unheard of in salamanders. A newfangled salvation, a newfangled salvaging of my sexuality and my sexual energies, a newfangled regeneration of my tail, my third leg.

Only with the greatest of humiliations does one have the opportunity to achieve a great comeback. The harder they fall, the harder they rise up. The hell with gravity.

CHAPTER 8

Oglia and Aglia

"No more pie now, no more crème brulee
Lay off the gravy and soufflé
No French fri-yi-yies now, No ice cream parfait
Mr. Cheese Nacho, Stay away."
     —Weird Al Yankovic, "Grapefruit Diet," a parody
              of "Zoot Suit Riot"

"A New Liquid Gold," or something to that effect, read the article in the science and technology section of *The Economist* in late 1984. I was looking for some new mantras, some new vows to sink my teeth into, and this article suggested that olive oil was it. Olio and aglia, olive oil and garlic, my new gods, my new objects of worship. I began to see how a religious fervor in the face of trichinosis or drinking problems can enhance the public health. Pork chops tasted too good to eliminate from the diet even in the face of widespread trichinosis. Alcohol was and is too wonderful a substance, not just in taste but in effect, to eliminate from the diet even in the face of widespread intoxication and debauchery. So, let's put doctrinal zeal into the mix, the laws of kashrut for Jews, the laws of hallal for Muslims.

Now a religion of one, my own doctrinal fervor, my own public health initiative—for a public of one solitary individual. Weirdly, the ideas have found me, not vice versa. Yet I am more open to new options and willing to consider alternative ways of eating. Like a baseball player who is hitting .150, I am more willing to listen to my batting instructor, to change my swing, to change my stance.

I grew up inadvertently and unadvisedly worshipping dead cows as part of a family legacy. Hindus, eat your hearts out. No chicken in every pot. No, a cow—a whole cow in every pot. The object of our family worship in childhood was an enormous freezer in our basement—a freezer with every kind of cow part imaginable, young cows and old cows, veal chops and veal flanks and steaks and brisket and hot dogs and chopped beef and corned beef and tongue and liver and sweetbreads and derma. The best beef that anyone could find.

My friends all had pool tables, ping-pong tables, televisions, and stereos in their basements. I had a freezer.

My grandfather, my mother's father, had set the stage for this animal-rich dietary tradition. He had come to America in 1892 from a tiny rural shtetl near the Russian-Polish border at the age of twelve. With the blessing of his parents, he arrived alone, a solitary figure, a mere child trying to avoid conscription in the Polish army. The oldest child in his family, he was their hope for a better future. Could he somehow make his way in America and eventually bring his parents and brothers and sisters to this country as well? A task he was more than able to achieve.

A not-too-atypical American immigrant story—except that, when he stepped off the boat, he had no idea where to go. All he knew was he did not want to spend a minute, let alone a lifetime, in New York City. The Lower East Side was not for this rural farm boy.

He hopped on a train at Grand Central Station without any clue where he was headed. When he was able to see he was in a rural enough area, he hopped off and started a new life, in Bridgeport, Connecticut. He had no urban skills. The only skill he knew was how to cut up cows and chickens. So he got a job working for a butcher. Within a couple of decades he had become the king of meat-wholesaling in Bridgeport. Even after he died when I was eight years old, my mother would still make biweekly trips from a town thirty miles away to pick up huge sides of beef from his company.

Like most children raised in the 1950s, I was nurtured and suckled on land animals. Vegetables were alien, except for some boiled canned peas to provide what my mother called a more balanced meal. I hated fish. Occasionally we would have a night of chicken or lamb chops, but we all knew that the dead cow was the one and only object of veneration.

Extra fatty dead cows. Among my friends and colleagues, I was well-known in my twenties and thirties for going into delicatessens and asking for extra fatty corned beef sandwiches. Still ringing in my ears are the words of my grandfather, reinforced by my father, "The more marbled and fatty the meat, the tastier it will be." A way of eating instilled in me when I was most suggestible. If we were not eating beef, we were all eating truckloads of cheeses and eggs and cream cheese and butter for breakfast.

So, why change a way of eating that was so hammered into me, a way of eating that may be impossible to change?

In the months after prostate surgery, I came across maps showing prostate cancer deaths around the world. In 1984, the highest death rates were in Switzerland and the United States, with the Scandinavian countries not far behind. Mediterranean countries had a somewhat lower death rate; and East Asia—particularly Japan and China—had an almost negligible death rate. Prostate cancer was a different disease in Asia, not nearly as aggressive and invasive. The disease, when it occurs, stays small and localized in the prostate, harmless and unobtrusive. Men in Asia, as of 1984, were truly dying *with* prostate cancer, not *of* prostate cancer.

Could it be just genes and genetic differences? Or was it the environment, or a different dietary pattern?

I knew enough about Switzerland to appreciate the ubiquity of their cows. The clanging of cowbells everywhere in the Alps during the summer months; the tomato soup with a dollop of cream so large you might as well call it cream soup with a touch of tomato; cheese, Swiss cheese of course, all around. Scandinavia, pretty much the same—a diet rich in meat and dairy products. When the data on prostate cancer deaths was collected in the previous quarter century, fruits and vegetables and olives and olive oil were not a staple of northern Europe. The easy transport of oils and greens from the south, or even from the southern hemisphere, was not up and running.

So too in the United States: The northern European diet ruled, especially in my family. Meat and potatoes, and dairy and more dairy.

Not so in Asia. Lactose intolerance, virtually everywhere in Asia, changed the rules of the game. No milk, no butter, no cream, no cheese. No dead cow in every pot as well. Few people in Asia had the resources to raise and kill and eat cows.

I had nothing to lose by changing my way of eating. I could not change my genes, but I could change my diet and my environment. I could also put myself to a test: could my newfound suggestibility and mantras allow me to change a highly engrained eating style?

No way was I going to turn to macrobiotics, as Anthony Satillaro had done. I had flirted with a macrobiotic diet, where you eat mostly grains, briefly in college and hated it. I tried it again very briefly, but brown rice did not rule; macrobiotic gruel did not rule. And I saw no evidence that a macrobiotic diet played any role in the low death rates from prostate cancer in Asia. The differences between the West and the East seemed simpler and more subtle than macrobiotic versus nonmacrobiotic.

So, I made some new vows: No dairy, no beef. Indeed "no land animals" whatsoever. Just fruits and vegetables, and loads of that liquid gold—olive oil. No butter on bread, instead olive oil. No blue cheese dressing on a salad, instead olive oil. No stir-fry with butter, only with olive oil. I was turning to the Mediterranean and Asia for my dietary inspiration, not to northern Europe and America.

Fortunately, I had grown up not only with beef and dairy but also with potatoes and peanut oil. My father had owned a large and successful potato chip company in Connecticut. I would skip school as often as possible and grab hot oily chips off the conveyor ramp after they had gone through the frying process. The oilier the bubbles in the chips, the better.

If our family was not busy worshipping dead cows, we were at least worshipping oil and potatoes. My father and I even used peanut oil from his factory to oil my baseball gloves, particularly my catcher's mitt, every spring. Nothing could have solidified my hypnotic connection with cooking oils more so than an idyllic potato chip factory and the bonding spring ritual of oiling my baseball gloves.

Dead cows are fine in the form of leather baseball gloves.

And then a new discovery for me in the fall of 1984: Peanut oil, like olive oil, is mostly a monounsaturated fat. Another liquid gold: potato chips and french fri-yi-yies. Yes, indeed. No more land animals, but peanut oil and olive oil will provide salvation.

And nuts as well—all kinds of nuts including almonds and cashews and the legume of peanuts. Nuts had been a close second to fries and chips as my favorite food. It helped that my father had been a distributor of Planters nuts at the same time he was producing and distributing his potato chips. So, pasta and stir-fried vegetables—in *oglio* and *aglia*—with plenty of fruits and nuts and chips and fries—a diet already more diverse and appealing than the diet of most Americans.

Yet, how does one give up ice cream and milk chocolate and cheeses? How does one overcome the indoctrination from earliest childhood about drinking four glasses of milk each day? How does one live with Oreo cookies without a glass of milk alongside?

Here Tony Robbins came to the rescue. While he put us into a hypnotic trance to walk across blisteringly hot coals, he reminded us that cow's milk was designed specifically for young calves—to help them grow into large cows. "Cow's milk is simply a substitute for human milk. Once we reach our adolescence, when our bones are fully formed and we are fully grown, there is no need for milk of any kind."

"It might be time to wean yourself off a cow's teat," he repeated several times. Having just read Toni Morrison's novel *Song of Solomon,* I could not stop thinking about "milkman," the young boy whose mother refused to wean him, the young boy who continued to breastfeed. Teased mercilessly by his peers and humiliated by the name "milkman," he provided a cautionary tale. How was I any different? A cow's teat, a goat's teat, a human teat: Am I not old enough at thirty-six to wean myself from a cow's teat, from any teat?

I began to see human disorders in a different light. How have we come to see lactose intolerance, a feature that affects 75 percent of the human population, as a disorder? A feature that develops in late adolescence, as if the food gods know that human beings need some powerful, negative reinforcement against drinking milk and eating concentrated milk in the form of cheese and against buttering our bread. These food gods are trying to protect us from heart disease and prostate cancer, but no one has been listening. Gas and diarrhea and abdominal pain have been delivering a message for several thousand years, a message mostly ignored.

A Eurocentric view of the world—yet it was only five or six thousand years ago that human beings living somewhere in England developed the capacity to tolerate lactose in adulthood. According to mappings of the human genome in 2002, scientists were able to trace lactose tolerance to a mutation in regulatory DNA that controls the lactase gene. Lactase, an enzyme in the intestines, allows infants and children, and now a sizable minority of adults, to digest a complex sugar in the form of lactose.

With this evolutionary development, people were able to move further and further north, from England on to the rest of northern Europe and to Scandinavia and even Iceland, where there were no greens, edible vegetables, or fruits for at least nine to ten months each year. Dairy was a lifesaver, the salvation for those migrating north. The herding of milk-producing animals became a way of life.

Likewise, in parts of East Africa and Saudi Arabia, where people traditionally herd milk-producing animals, a different mutation affecting the same gene developed to help herders and their families tolerate lactose. Culture can indeed reinforce the forces of evolution.

So, I began to create my own culture, my own evolutionary forces. I mutated from someone who combined the worst of the Swiss and Scandinavian and American diets into someone who now has forsaken everything related to land animals. I forsake the milk from their breasts; I forsake the flesh from their corpses.

In the 1990s a report came out in the *New England Journal of Medicine* indicating that a substance called oleo-linoleic acid is a crucial factor in the development of aggressive prostate cancer. This form of linoleic acid is found only in . . . land animals. So what if the report was premature, and the findings did not pan out. My religion of one did not allow for doubt.

Some new mantras were forming: I have gleaned enough to be weaned; I am keen to be clean of land animals; I will no longer allow myself to be seen as a conventional "milkman." Screw those old dietary conventions.

Then George Sheehan came along to reinforce my new belief system. A runner and a cardiologist and a writer, he had just been diagnosed with prostate cancer—and later died of it in 1993. He similarly had changed his diet, not so much to prevent the prostate cancer from becoming more aggressive, but to prevent his dying from some other more acute disease. No heart attacks, no strokes, or CVAs (cerebral vascular accidents), no adult-onset diabetes for him, thank you very much.

Another mantra: I want to live long enough to die *of* prostate cancer, not *with* prostate cancer. I want to die via a slow boil, a death indeed on the installment plan. No quick untimely death allowed.

Yes, the horses have already escaped from the barn; the disease was already in full flower. Was there any logic in closing the barn door at this point? Perhaps fatty acids from land animals might be instrumental in making the disease more aggressive and invasive, I thought. I had nothing to lose in trying to rein in those horses and those fatty acids.

This was my first test after the diagnosis of prostate cancer. Could I evolve? Could I mutate in response to these new cultural and medical demands? Could my mind have a mind of its own? I had some newfound missionary zeal. But my custom-made religion of one and by one and for one was not a fundamentalist creed: I encouraged my family, my disciples, to eat plenty of cheese and other dairy products in their younger years, and unsuccessfully tried to convince my daughters that a childhood and adolescence without a few corned beef sandwiches is a hopelessly deprived one. They could cut back on dairy and meat later in their adult lives.

This religion now has its own slogans and rallying cries. "No ice cream parfaits, no MIs no CVAs, no crème brulée—cheese nachos, stay away."

I have my own prayer or vow, bizarre and paradoxical as any prayer can be: "Let me die *of* prostate cancer, and do not let me die of some other more acute disease, or any disease associated with the typical American diet. As a mere mortal I wish to live long enough to have prostate cancer kill me."

I had the symbols of my faith: olive oil and peanut oil, potato chips and French fries, with more than a little broccoli and other cruciferous vegetables thrown in for good measure.

I can think of worse things to worship.

CHAPTER 9

Oxygen—and A Cannot-Do Philosophy

". . . there are places in this world where the safety net they (Westerners) have spent so much of their lives erecting is suddenly whipped away, where the right accent, education, health insurance and a foreign passport . . . no longer apply, and their well-being depends on the condescension of strangers."

—Michela Wrong, *In the Footsteps of Mr. Kurtz: Living on the Brink of Disaster in the Congo*

It pays to be deluded.

As a psychiatrist I am well aware of the fact that people who are depressed have a better handle on reality than people who are not depressed. The depressed person has a fuller grasp of his own mortality, of the morbidities of life, of the futility and fruitlessness of existence, of the wisdom of John Maynard Keynes's line that in the long run we are all dead.

At the same time, I grew up in 1950s America, with a can-do philosophy that for every problem there is a solution. We had the buoyancy from the war, and our self-assuredness from having beaten the Nazis and the militaristic Japanese, and we had by far the best educational system in the world that excluded no one. We had the rags-to-riches stories of Horatio Alger to inspire us in this optimistic and empowering view of life.

It pays to believe fancifully that obstacles are opportunities, to forget that obstacles are truly obstacles.

But it also pays to be aware of our screwups, to accommodate the yin and the yang, to allow for doubts and misgivings along with answers and fixes. Often the fixes come only through screwups, particularly when it comes to potential antidotes and fixes for the effects of radiation treatment.

So, praise the old Soviets. The Soviet Union unwittingly provided the experimental subjects for radiation meltdowns, radiation accidents, radiation explosions—all leading to radiation sickness and to thyroid diseases and to blood dyscrasias and to radiation deaths. Praise to the old Soviets for insisting on keeping these meltdowns and explosions secret so that the experiences could be repeated over and over and over again. When scientific journal articles suggest in their conclusions that some of the data and findings may need to be replicated, they were preaching to the choir in the Soviet Union. The Soviet findings invariably got replicated—and confirmed.

So, by early 1985 when I was going through thirty or more days of radiation to the prostate bed, I was aware of a growing body of knowledge coming out in bits and pieces from Russia. Chernobyl in April 1986, was the most publicized radiation event in the Soviet bloc and forced the Soviet Union to abandon its secrecy—but that event was thirteen months after the end of my radiation. A major accident occurred in 1957 in the east Urals in the development and use of plutonium for bomb development. But this event—despite its widespread destruction and devastation—was kept secret for thirty years. In the 1980s, at the time of my exposure to radiation, news was dribbling out about smaller events near the Poland-Russia border— accidents that affected radiation plant workers but not local civilians.

Sigmund Freud once noted that he learned the most about psychiatric treatment when he lost a patient who left therapy abruptly because of a mistake he had made. If we never screw up, we then never develop new skills or new ways of understanding the world.

The Soviet radiation workers gave us some wonderful gifts in the midst of their suffering and dying. They taught us how radiation kills living cells. And the Soviet government, desperate to keep these disasters secret, looked urgently for antidotes to radiation exposure—better to keep the masses quiet.

The yin needs the yang, the can-dos need the cannot-dos, the maturing fragrant flowers need the reeking manure, matter needs antimatter, the facile need the screwups. And the capitalists need the communists.

The Russians confirmed that radiation takes its destructive action in a variety of ways. First photons—elementary particles that have characteristics of both particles and waves and are a "unit" of light—penetrate the protoplasm of one's living cells. These photons interact with the protoplasm to create ion pairs, which in turn react radiochemically with water (H_2O) to produce hydroxyl (OH) and hydrogen (H) free radicals. These free radicals produce a further chain of reactions, creating new reactive forms, lasting only millionths of a second, like hydrogen peroxide (H_2O_2) and hydrogen dioxide (HO_2) and trihydrogen oxide (H_3O)—weird stuff instead of water. In rapid succession these odd and contrived products react with critical protoplasmic molecules in DNA and in enzymes. Cells either die precipitously, or at best they are unable to divide and proliferate in their normal fashion. Approximately two-thirds of the radiation damage to DNA in mammalian cells is caused by hydroxyl (OH) radicals.

Some other less understood degenerative processes may occur in brain and neural tissue. Radiation may cause a demyelination of the nerve fibers. In a process not unlike that which occurs in multiple sclerosis, the fibers lose their myelin sheaths—sheaths that are essential for the conduction of electrical charges and signals.

Hyperbaric oxygen, the Russians discovered, is an antidote to many of these radiation phenomena. The inhalation of oxygen at high pressure forces oxygen into tissues and cells, which, after exposure to radiation, are starving for oxygen and its life-giving power. This heavy infusion of oxygen may reverse the processes unleashed by radiation and may allow barely viable cells—cells dormant and on the verge of a final death—to come back to life.

Hyperbaric oxygen was well-known for years as a singular and necessary treatment for decompression sickness. If a diver is decompressing too abruptly during a deep-sea dive, in his rising too quickly to the surface, the blood vessels become permeated with nitrogen bubbles that interfere with the natural perfusion of oxygen into cells and tissue. Just as oxygen delivered at high atmospheric pressure rids the body of these nitrogen-bubble toxins, this same oxygen, the Russians discovered, may push out the toxic effects of radiation.

As I was going through my own exposure to toxic amounts of radiation, word was coming out that the Russians had some impressive results in using hyperbaric oxygen chambers for their exposed radiation workers.

I filed this information away and jumped into action during the summer. I had my mantra of doing everything I could to restore my sexual health, my new way of eating, and my own surprise and encouragement that I had been able to abide by it. I also had intense motivation, fueled by desolation and despair.

I called around the Washington, DC, area to find out who was offering hyperbaric oxygen treatments. One large chamber at a university hospital in Baltimore was too cumbersome a drive for daily treatments for four weeks. Another program was in a small community hospital in northern Virginia, in Mount Vernon near George Washington's home and close to what is now called Reagan National Airport. The two glass-enclosed chambers in a tiny room catered to divers with the bends, who were flown up to National Airport from naval stations in Portsmouth and Newport News, Virginia, and occasional recreational divers fresh from calamities in the Caribbean, with a few rare gas-gangrene cases and suicidal patients poisoned by carbon monoxide through a car exhaust thrown in.

The medical director of this small unit was itching for some new targets for his interventions. A 1960s Marlboro man now in his fifties—fortunately he snuffed out his cigarettes before going anywhere near the oxygen chambers—he was intrigued by my idea that high concentrations of oxygen would be the ideal antidote for my sexual wreckage. He seemed to feel my pain and identify with the horror of losing one's sexual capacities at age thirty-six. Not unlike me he had read the literature describing what the Russians had been doing to assist their wounded workers. My being a physician seemed to help my case. He perceived me as a reasonable guy, not a quack. Looks can deceive.

A man of few words, the Marlboro man said, "Let's give it a try. We have nothing to lose."

It pays to be lucky. My health insurance fully covered this treatment. Long before the advent of managed care in the early nineties, we were living in the mid-eighties, when physician recommendations ruled. My Marlboro man told the insurance company I would benefit from this treatment, and the insurance company went along with it.

Ah, the good old days. Days when the psychiatrist and *Washington Post* columnist Charles Krauthammer received extensive long-term treatment and support for his quadriplegia, suffered after a ruinous swimming pool accident while in medical school. The hospital care and institutional support allowed him to complete medical school, a psychiatry residency, a National Institutes of Health (NIH) fellowship, and move on to his life as a writer.

I was merely looking to get erect.

—∞—

The hyperbaric oxygen treatments worked—at least temporarily. I went through twenty consecutive treatments, five to six each week, two hours each. After about thirteen or fourteen treatments, I felt some stirrings in my pelvis. Nothing grand, nothing dramatic, but some miniscule partial erections in the mornings. I was ecstatic. Some cells were still alive. Not all the tissue in the pelvis had become necrotic and scarred; some dormant cells on the verge of dying were perhaps being brought back to life.

By the twentieth and final treatment, what was miniscule was now more erect—not a full erection but at least workable. Helen and I were able to have sex, not great sex, but immeasurably better than nothing. Yes, the joy, the over-joy, of sex. When we lose something essential and then regain it—oh man, what a joy, not to be taken for granted ever again.

This vow, this mantra was already paying dividends. This effort was easier and the rewards faster than anyone could have predicted.

Ah, not so fast: The outcome did not last. I lost my erections. A week or two after the conclusion of the twenty treatments, the gains dissolved. A psychic deflation following my erectile inflation.

"How 'bout we try it again, doc?"

"Sure, why not?" the doc muttered with a cigarette hanging from his lips.

Twenty more treatments—the same result. Initial inflation followed by debilitating deflation. Modest erections, then nada. Twenty more treatments, then twenty more. This guy at Mount Vernon Hospital truly felt my pain. Short-term gains, no long-term ones, though.

Eighty treatments in, we gave up. I could not spend the rest of my life in a hyperbaric chamber.

My spin: My efforts could be rewarded. Keep pushing, keep trying. Not too picturesque, but it was picaresque, nevertheless. A new kind of quest, an inner pursuit—no traveling the Mississippi in a raft, no traveling through a heart of darkness in the Congo—instead a penile and mental and emotional quest, a quest of the inner life with every neuron in my body engaged, especially every neuron in my brain and my pelvis.

The salamander had not quite regenerated its tail, but oxygen had brought new life, temporarily, and renewed hope to my own tail.

CHAPTER 10

The Infertile Road to Chinese Medicine: A Better Life Through Electricity, Not Chemistry

"The art of healing is thousands of years old. The science of healing is still in the process of being born."
—David Eisenberg, *Encounters with Qi*

"The methods used by one man may be faulty; the methods used by two men will be better."
—Chinese Proverb

"Illness is comparable to the root . . . If the root is not reached, the evil influences cannot be subjugated."
—Traditional Chinese Medicine Texts

"Haughtiness invites ruin; humility receives benefits."
—The Chinese *Book of Changes*

Libido, yes; potency, no. And fertility? None. What is going on here? In a biblical sense, what is the point of fucking?

I was dry humping as best I could. Dry, no ejaculant, but my testicles were producing sperm. No one cut into or cut off my balls. I was thirty-six years old, Helen was thirty-five—right in the heart of her reproductive years. We always wanted a third child and now this was thwarted.

A lack of fertility cuts right into our basic raison d'etre. It is automatic, it is instinctual, it is reflexive, it is unconscious and unmeditated. Our instincts tell us: reproduce, breed and spawn and regenerate; ensure the survival of our species, of our people, of each and every one of our genes. Our texts tell us: be fruitful and multiply.

Yet childless couples are more contented and happier in their fifties and sixties than couples with children in the same cohort. So much for reflexes and instincts.

And yet . . . the term "maternal instincts" may have been coined with Helen in mind. At his primate lab at the National Institutes of Health in Poolesville, Maryland, Stephen Suomi has described some primate mothers as being "super-mothers." They have just the right touch; they are rarely punitive with their offspring. Even when matched with baby monkeys who are skittish and sensitive by temperament, these super-mothers provide a loving and caring environment that allows these babies and youngsters to explore their world in bold and courageous ways.

Helen fit the bill.

So, what had I been thinking? Where was my head? Up my ass, worrying about potency, penetration, penis, pelvis. What about Helen, what about fertility, and our having a third child? Yes, we had two wonderful daughters. We had not been infertile from the get-go. No reason to feel sorry for Helen or for the two of us. Yet it was hard to see a talent stopped in its tracks just as it was reaching its prime—not unlike an athlete stopped in his tracks by a leg injury or a concussion, not unlike a pianist or violinist who can no longer use his hands, not unlike a chef who loses his sense of smell and taste.

I got on the horn with the prostate surgeon at Columbia-Presbyterian Medical Center. "Okay, so we never collected any sperm before the surgery. But what can I do now? How do I regain some semblance of fertility?"

"We can extract sperm from your testes. The sperm should be viable. There's a guy I know well at an academic medical center in Houston who can extract the sperm. He's a nationally recognized fertility expert. He can do a needle biopsy. I'll call him today and see what we can arrange."

Doctor talk for, "We'll put a large needle in one of your balls and see what we find."

Oh, fuck. Ow, ouch. A new way of fucking, a new way of making babies. A new kind of intimacy.

Within days I was in an operating room in Houston undergoing this needle biopsy. I must have been in a hell of a trance. My vows, my mantras were taking me to strange places—this trip to Houston, this enthusiasm for putting my testicles under the knife. Was this my plan, or some master plan designed by Aristophanes? Potency will wait; fertility comes first.

A few days later, back in Washington, DC, I heard from the fertility guy. "Your sperm cells have been affected by the radiation. They are extremely immature and currently unviable. That could change in the next few months or years. Let's keep in touch. We can do the same procedure down the road."

What had Helen and I been thinking? Of course the radiation had a profound effect on rapidly reproducing cells like sperm cells. The fertility guy had seen only what was visible under the microscope. What about the invisible effects of radiation? Radiation scientists speak of "bad invisible information"—information stored in proliferative cells, in the DNA. This faulty coding can lead to congenital and degenerative diseases in the bone marrow and elsewhere—untold consequences on any offspring. Visions of a child with two heads and one arm and three legs come to mind.

Here is what Eric Hall, the author of the definitive textbook on radiobiology, has to say about radiation damage, "If the damage is a mutation in a germ cell leading to hereditary changes, it may not be expressed for many generations." What a legacy—great-great-grandchildren with two heads. Thank the gods for immature and unviable sperm—at least no legacy of horrors three or four generations from now.

An unusual mourning dawned on Helen and me, a mourning over an ambiguous loss. No, this was not the sense of loss one feels after a miscarriage or after a stillbirth or after the death of a young child. This was a grief over all the unborn children, over all of what might have transpired, over all of the abstract potential for life, all of it intangible and unpalpable. No remains, no coffins, no ashes, no stones to mark the grave, no tombs to mark the loss. No religious institution or rituals to grab onto. No ceremonies, no funeral services, no wakes—no priest or rabbi to mark this loss of fertility, this end of a couple's unique gift, a gift for themselves and from themselves to the world.

No wonder then, in all species except man—and man only in the last century—life expectancy coincides with the age of male or female menopause. A question from the gods: Is there any point to life after our reproductive years have ended? Finality and the end of fertility—one and the same, say the gods of ontogeny and phylogeny.

Helen and I fortunately still had two young daughters, then five and seven years old, to raise—a genuine life's work and pleasure, a reason to live beyond one's end of fertility.

Plus we had a new torment to confront.

—⁓—

Oh, fuck. I had unremitting and unrelenting pain in my left testicle ever since the surgeon stuck a needle into it. The area healed uneventfully, but the pain never stopped. My pelvis seemed to be a tinderbox, neurally ready to explode, with sensory fibers confused and overloaded and unable to figure out what they were connected to.

The surgeon in Houston had never seen such a response to a "simple" needle biopsy. Simple, my ass. Simple, my balls.

It appeared to be some kind of causalgia or neuralgia, according to the terminology of 1985. People can get these causalgias in the brachial plexus above the shoulder—causing horrific pain in the arms. Others can suffer from a similar phenomenon in the sciatic nerve in the lower back. Still others, having gone through an amputation of a limb, can have an unremitting phantom-limb pain. But how many people end up with an unrelenting pain in the balls? Or in one ball to be exact—one ball too many.

Neurology textbooks at the time described causalgia as a "distressing symptom," a hell of an understatement. Lord Brain, the aptly named writer of the definitive neurology textbook used in 1985, described it as an "intense and persistent burning pain, which is subject to paroxysmal exacerbations, which may be excited . . . by actual contact with the (affected) limb." Yeah, my limb, my tail, my testicle was simply getting the wrong kind of excitement.

The treatments for this condition, circa 1985, were ghastly and mostly ineffective. Surgeons had to resort to a sympathectomy, the cutting of the damaged peripheral nerve that was the source of the pain and the cutting of the sympathetic nervous system stimulation in the area. But in an area dense with neural tissue, how can anyone know which of the many peripheral nerves is implicated?

No one was going near my balls, if I had a say. No scalpels, no needles, no medical palpations. I was already relentless in second-guessing the original needle biopsy. Relentless pain and relentless second-guessing.

Then I had physicians stating or implying the pain must be all in my head, that it cannot possibly be real. The pain was unimaginable—no one could conceive of it. Proof positive of Philip Roth's notion, "Nothing that befalls anyone is too senseless to have happened." Proof positive of Susan Sontag's notion: The default assumption surrounding any mysterious ailment, a problem without a known clear-cut cause, is that it is "all psychological."

I envisioned myself rotting in a revolving door of chronic-pain-clinic hell, a torture that might be worse than the actual pain.

—⁂—

Into this void stepped a surprising figure—my internist. A conventional guy, thorough and systematic in his approach to patients, standing behind a veneer of scientific detachment, he oddly suggested I try acupuncture and sent me over to Jing Wu.

Wu turned out to be a more than fascinating fellow. He was living proof of the absurdity of F. Scott Fitzgerald's line that "there are no second acts in American lives." Here Wu was in his second act, after having been run out of Wall Street by the Securities and Exchange Commission (SEC) in his initial career as an investment banker. With a financial scandal behind him, with the loss of millions of dollars—when that sum meant something—Wu had no choice but to reinvent himself.

He turned back to his Chinese roots, to his roots growing up above his parents' laundry in Greenwich, Connecticut, and used his Harvard education and considerable intellectual curiosity and energy to understand the vagaries of Chinese medicine. Without any formal education in anything remotely connected to clinical medicine, Western or Eastern, he arranged apprenticeships over the years with Chinese medicine experts in Hong Kong and on the Chinese mainland. He was a throwback to the way careers developed in previous centuries, when people developed skills as farmers and artisans and even potato chip makers through apprenticeships, not through college and graduate school educations.

He could talk about fire and water, the kidney pulse, the spleen pulse, now with the best of them in China and the United States—all mumbo jumbo to anyone with a Western-trained ear.

Wu threw himself into his second act. He took on the task of coming up with a new translation of the *I Ching*, otherwise known as the Chinese *Book of Changes*, which explored the dynamic balance between opposites. A newly-minted Daoist, he put together a new translation of Lao Tsu's *Tao Te Ching*, a series of poems and statements that looks at the paradoxes of life while preaching humility and a willingness to go with the flow.

A remarkable second act, though a bit more subdued than his first. In his first act he was purported to have had an affair with Jacqueline Kennedy Onassis when she lived in a home he owned in Middleburg, Virginia.

In his second act, he reinvented himself in the image of a traditional Chinese peasant doctor.

—∞—

Wu's intervention worked, and worked almost immediately. In my first encounter with him, he delicately put needles into my back, mostly in the lumbosacral region.

"We want to find a way for the brain, the leader of the nervous system, to believe that the radiated and scarred tissue in the prostate bed is still viable and alive. It is as if your brain has written off that area of the body, has assumed it is all dead and desolate—and your brain is now receiving weird and distorted signals from that part of the body."

My pelvis had become some fallow acreage, not worthy of any irrigation or seeding or cultivation. Wu and I wanted to find some way to reverse the brain's perception.

There is nothing like quick success to make us into converts. Religion is notorious for producing a similar quick conversion. Nostalgia for our childhood innocence, when the world seemed simpler and safer, can lead us back to religion in our grimmest and grimiest hours. It works almost immediately; it provides instant comfort—and we are hooked, born-again Christians, Muslims, Jews before we know what hit us.

Acupuncture is a harder sell, especially in the West in 1985 and 1986. Even the Chinese themselves had forgotten and neglected this cultural and medical treasure over the preceding hundred years. In the late nineteenth and for the first half of the twentieth century, Western medicine in China was in unprecedented ascendancy, and traditional Chinese medicine was in unprecedented descendency. The medical teaching programs initiated in China by Western institutions such as Harvard, Yale, and the Rockefeller Foundation were exceeded only by the highly Westernized medical school developed by St. John's University in Shanghai in the late nineteenth century. By the time the Nationalist government of Chiang Kai-Shek came along, leaders were more than willing to sell traditional Chinese medicine down the proverbial Yangtze River. In fact, the government passed legislation to outlaw traditional medical approaches like acupuncture and herbs on the grounds that it was backward and primitive and laden with superstition.

Under Mao Zedong the communists took a more pragmatic, albeit cynical, approach. "We have an enormous country, with only thirty-eight thousand Western-trained doctors serving five hundred million people," they seemed to be saying. "Let's throw the population a bone by hurling three hundred thousand traditional medicine specialists at them to give some semblance of providing for their medical needs."

Mao did initiate some notable public health and preventative medicine campaigns. But the situation took a major turn for the worse with the Cultural Revolution in 1965. During the first six years of this revolting revolution, all medical schools, including schools of traditional medicine, were closed. When they reopened, their curricula were decimated along with any pretense of a meritocracy. Students were not selected for admission based on their capabilities, but instead on vague political considerations like a "willingness to serve the people." No cynic could have devised a more dramatic means for destroying a rich medical tradition—a distinct and complementary view of how the human body operates, compared to the West—than Mao and the Gang of Four and their predecessors had done.

Only in 1976, with the death of Mao and the overthrow of the Gang of Four, did traditional Chinese medicine begin to make a comeback. But that comeback would take a number of years to spill over into the West.

So, acupuncture in 1985, in Washington, DC, had little or no cachet. But for me the second treatment worked even better than the first. The ungodly pain in my testicle was receding, and it was being replaced by a more appropriate and understandable pain in my lower pelvis, at the site of the scarring from the surgery and radiation.

This evolving pain, I could handle. Exercise, exercise, exercise: Basketball and tennis became my daily staple. But the pain became exacerbated with any effort to move the muscles of the pelvis, with any pelvic thrust or pelvic tilt. When squeezing in and tightening these pelvic muscles—something we naturally do when holding in a bowel movement, or when getting sexually aroused—I could feel a burning and knife-like sensation in the lower pelvis.

"The normal muscle tissue is trying to push and pull and contract alongside the really scarred and unmovable tissue," Wu explained. "When you squeeze in, the burned and radiated tissue remains stuck, glued to its bony insertions. The normal muscles are out-of-sync with this fixed and rigid scarred stuff.

"At some point after we convince your brain to pay attention to this scarred stuff, to recognize that this dead detritus is worthy of nourishment, we'll tackle the scarred tissue directly." For the first six months, Wu put needles exclusively in my back, in the intervertebral spaces, as I lie on my stomach.

Months later as I lay on my back, he put needles directly into the scar tissue in my lower abdomen. "The needles produce a histaminic effect," he noted confidently, "not unlike a mosquito bite.

Each needle insertion is like a mini-surgery that activates a healing response from the body. With this little prick—no pun intended—your blood stream goes into action. Your red cells, your white cells gravitate to the area of this tiny, tiny injury. If we tried to break up the scar tissue with a scalpel, we would simply be wreaking more havoc and creating more scar tissue. With these tiny needles we may even be inducing the creation of new blood vessels that can then perfuse this heavily scarred tissue. We're creating new canals, new conduits to nourish this decaying tissue."

A new image took hold—scarred, hard brown tissue becoming pink and soft, well oxygenated and revascularized. A mantra came with it: I will do everything I can to bring these pelvic cells back to life, to make them pink and soft. Pink and purple, those colors again, reflecting verve and vibrancy. With each treatment the discomfort in my pelvis was changing ever so slightly, and the pain in the left testicle was gone forever.

I have become a convert, a true believer. The relief of torture will do that to you.

—⊷—

No one knows definitively how acupuncture works. For musculoskeletal problems it works just as well on animals as it does on people. In 1986 as I was continuing acupuncture treatments, I came across research from A. M. Schoen showing that acupuncture relieves symptoms and increases activity in 80 percent of animals with degenerative joint disease—disease previously unresponsive to conventional treatments. X-rays of the involved joints before and after treatment suggest some regeneration in the damaged joint cartilage.

Others are more dismissive, claiming that acupuncture simply activates a placebo response. "If you believe it, it will come." In essence, they are saying it is purely a psychological response, not a physical one. Again Susan Sontag's point: When phenomena are poorly understood, we apply psychological reasoning—it is all in the person's head—to explain both poorly understood illnesses as well as poorly understood healing experiences.

If it is a placebo, I am going for it. Let's bottle it and use it and benefit from it.

Wu and other traditional Chinese practitioners did not help their case with their narratives and language. Twelve meridians or channels, fifteen collaterals, eight extra channels, and hundreds of acupuncture points defined by these channels and collaterals. My eyes glazed over as Wu described the five basic elements from which the universe and man himself is made—wood, earth, water, fire, and metal.

"Each organ of the body corresponds to one of the elements," Wu pointed out. "For example, the liver corresponds to wood, and the heart corresponds to fire. Each of the five elements is a subdivision of yin and yang: The solid organs are considered yin while the hollow organs, like the intestines, are considered yang."

Okay . . .

And then the feeling of the radial pulse. We Western-trained doctors feel the pulse to determine how the heart is functioning: Is the pulse too fast or too slow, are there irregular beats, is the strength of the pulse too thready? The Chinese peasant doctor feels different kinds of pulses over the course of one centimeter of the radial artery along the wrist. These pulsations, they claim, may reflect imbalances in, say, the liver or kidney, not just the heart.

Wu reminded me all the time that my kidney pulse was quite weak. This kidney pulse reflects the energy level along the kidney meridian controlling sexual function and activity. No surprise there.

The simplicity of this approach may be half its appeal. Just feel the pulse and examine the tongue—a more primitive and personal approach to medical care. No hammerings of the magnetic resonance imaging, no excessive and unnecessary radiation from CAT (CT) scans, no ultrasounds, no blood tests.

So, how did acupuncture develop 5,000 years ago, with metal needles coming into play 2,300 years ago? Surely not by trial and error. One would have to take guinea pig status to absurd levels to imagine a host of human beings willing to let a crazed needle-wielder put hundreds of needles all over their bodies in an effort to see which points were useful.

The best clue may come from the Wang sisters. David Eisenberg in his book *Encounters with Qi* describes his remarkable encounter with these two young girls. They could describe in exquisite detail what was written on a piece of paper inside a closed box without previously having set eyes on the box or on the paper. They could even tell the color of the ink used on the paper. To Eisenberg's amazement these seemingly ordinary girls were able to repeat this feat easily in front of Eisenberg and several other Western physicians. The girls could also "see the outline of internal organs simply by looking at a patient's body . . . could determine the hair length and sex of an unborn fetus by inspecting the abdomen of a pregnant woman."

These girls had not recognized the uniqueness of their talent until their father had mentioned over dinner a newspaper story about a Sichuan boy who had similar capabilities. They had assumed everyone could do what they could do; they took it for granted. Chinese historians and researchers who have looked at this phenomenon have come to believe that these "exceptional human body functions" are inborn in a rare child, perhaps one in several million. Fortunately for the rest of humanity, the Chinese have admired and cultivated these exceptional capabilities through Qi Gong and acupuncture rather than letting them wither and die.

How many one-in-a-million clairvoyants and telepathic superstars has the Western world failed to nurture, out of our own ignorance and arrogance?

The unseeable, the unknowable: The Wang sisters may have had a special power enabling them to manipulate electrical currents and energy, what the Chinese call Qi. We here in the West have focused almost exclusively on chemical manipulations, not electrical interventions. Better living through chemistry—not a bad way to go, given the power of antibiotics to resolve infections, the power of antidepressants to stabilize mood. Yes, nerve impulses are propagated by neurotransmitters, and we in the West have figured out how to manipulate serotonin and dopamine and adrenaline levels, all to enormous advantage.

But the yin needs the yang. A solo ride on the back of chemistry leaves out energy and electricity. How might our chemical manipulations alter our electrical impulses at the synaptic level? For example, how might our chemical interventions, our medications like the simple element or cation lithium manipulate and change energy levels in a disorder like manic-depressive illness that is as much an energy disturbance as it is a mood disturbance?

Is there a way to imagine a better living through electrical gradients?

Yes, indeed. The salamander remains my model—again, the only vertebrate that can regenerate its foreleg, its hind leg, eye, ear, as much as one-third of its brain, almost all of its digestive tract, and up to one half of its heart. Astounding—and even more astounding is the fact that the next animal up on the evolutionary scale, the frog, has lost this capacity for regeneration. We humans can regenerate bone after a fracture and skin after a cut—and that is our limit in restorative returns. For frogs and humans, fibrosis and scarring are the order of the day.

When we look at the electrical currents and voltages at the amputation sites of salamanders versus frogs, the difference is striking. The direction of current at the injury site is diametrically opposite in these two closely related species. In the salamander, the current of injury is negative, unlike the positive current of injury in the frog. Indeed the control system that starts and regulates and stops healing in living bodies is electrical, not just chemical.

A frog's cells can be made regeneration-ready by simple exposure to astonishingly low levels of electricity measured in billionths of amperes. But even with this electrical manipulation, the frog is limited in its ability to regenerate by its small number of cells that can dedifferentiate, that can regress into primitive embryonic cells that can later differentiate into complex nerve and blood and muscle and bone cells.

Acupuncture may be one of the only human interventions that can create a negative polarity at a wound site. The insertion of a metal needle into the skin produces a tiny electrical current, and the miniscule injury from the needle entry is nevertheless large enough to create a local current of injury. A twisting of the needle may also produce a pulsing current at a low frequency.

Somehow, some wunderkinds not unlike the Wang sisters intuitively figured out these currents, these meridians and channels five thousand years ago.

I was determined to imagine a world in which there was better living through electrical currents and gradients. I realized I was no better off than the frog; I had a limited capacity to produce primitive dedifferentiated cells after the insults of surgery and radiation. All I could attempt to do was maximize the number of these cells and optimize the development of them—to see if they could evolve into highly differentiated nerve cells and blood vessel cells and muscle cells, and see if paralyzing fibrous scar tissue could turn into reasonably healthy and functioning neural and muscle tissue.

Little did I know at the time that this effort was going to take on a long and protracted course. No wonder Western medical practices have focused on chemical cures and modulating medications. The magic bullet works quickly and expeditiously. The alternative Eastern approach is a journey seemingly without end; the Western approach is a hurried destination.

Sisyphus was no longer a myth for me. He and his myth had become my reality.

CHAPTER 11

A Funny Thing Happened on the Way Back to Potency

"Comedy is simply tragedy plus time."
　　　　　　　—Unknown (often Attributed to Mark
　　　　　　　　　　　　Twain or Carol Burnett)

Cancer is a number of powers mightier than a wart.

My friends and colleagues started sending me journal articles with well-designed studies noting that visualization could help rid the body of warts and other minor viral maladies. Visualization techniques could also manipulate the extent of an inflammatory response after a cut or laceration. Through visualization we could, almost miraculously, either increase the inflammatory response or diminish it.

Ah, the powers of the human mind—a beautiful thing to contemplate. Let's party, let's celebrate, let's rejoice at the wonders of the human spirit, let's praise man's capacity to recover and regenerate. Prostate cancer was beating a hasty retreat, and my mind was working wonders on my body.

It was October 1989, five exact years since diagnosis and initial surgical treatment. I was feeling damned good. The surgeons kept reminding me that they had gotten it all, and for good measure we had killed any wayward cancer cells with 6600 rads of radiation.

No signs of recurrence. Plus, I had managed to defy the laws of nature by re-establishing some modicum of potency and sexual functioning, with the promise of more to come.

I was continuing with regular acupuncture, having learned to administer the needles myself, with the help of Jing Wu. Monkey see, monkey do—needles into the scar tissue of the lower abdomen and pelvis to help break up that scar tissue. Magnificent visualizations of my magenta, my pink and my purple immune cells grabbing and dismantling any black and yellow fly-like cancer cells in my Venus flytrap apparatus. Magnificent visualizations of the hardened brown scar tissue becoming pink and pliable and perfused. Magnificent experiences of sex with Helen, my libido and lust as strong as ever.

W. H. Auden again: "Lust is less a physical need than a way of forgetting time and death." I had forgotten time and death. I was in the moment, and moment after moment was magnificent.

My swagger was back. Prowess and pluck and pride were words I became reacquainted with. I left the University of Maryland to become associate director of the newly redesigned Georgetown University Counseling and Psychiatric Service, and I reassured my new colleagues and employers that I was healthy, having recovered from my "bout" with prostate cancer. My cancer had not been a secret. I had written about it in the newly established health section of the *Washington Post*, and Helen and I had been the subject of a profile on the "sandwich generation" in the local glossy *Washingtonian* magazine a few months prior—with reflections on our aging parents and our young children and my own health problems.

Everything seemed to be in sync.

Except, there were some flies in the ointment. The Venus flytrap had not been able to catch all the flies.

In December 1989, the surgeon in Manhattan called me a few weeks after our regular yearly follow-up appointment.

"Your PSA is rising," he soberly told me.

"What the hell is a PSA?"

"This is a new test, the prostate-specific antigen, something we can detect in the bloodstream. We've been experimenting with its use here. We didn't tell you at the time, but we've been measuring your PSA for the past two years. In December 1987, two years ago, your PSA was undetectable. Last December it had risen to 0.6, a borderline figure that could possibly have represented a recurrence. But since the test is so new, we didn't know how to interpret it, and I didn't want to scare you unnecessarily. But now the PSA is 2.1. Since you have no prostate, you shouldn't have any prostate activity anywhere in your body."

He could have added, but he did not, "So, now it's time to scare you."

"Isn't it possible that these are normal prostate cancer cells that have come back to life?" I asked, hopeful, thinking all too bizarrely and optimistically that my visualizations and acupuncture created some immaculate conceptions. Denial is a beautiful thing. In this case it did not last for long.

"No. No chance of that."

When these surgeons said they got it all, doubt never entered the picture—even when they did not get it all.

"I want you to come up to New York. We'll put you under general anesthesia and look in the area where the prostate used to be and see if we can find any palpable evidence of the cancer. We can always re-treat if we find the cancer cells in the prostate bed." Little did he or I know at the time that a PSA of 2.1 generally meant microscopic cancer disease, not something that would be visible in a surgical observation. Again, in 1989, no one seemed to have a clue on how to interpret the PSA.

He insisted, based on the scientific literature that early intervention for metastatic prostate cancer was crucial.

Yeah, early intervention—a euphemism for surgical castration—the cutting off of my balls. All that effort to save my potency, to save my pelvis, to save my life as a man—all down the drain.

I knew enough from medical school to recognize that the only treatment available for metastatic prostate cancer that has spread systemically to lymph nodes and bones and into the bloodstream and beyond the prostate, was castration. In 1941 Charles Huggins and Clarence V. Hodges discovered that prostate cancer growth could be slowed or in some cases eliminated by the removal of testosterone. Male hormones, otherwise known as androgens, were a crucial growth factor for prostate cancer. Androgen deprivation could stop prostate cancer in its tracks, at least temporarily. Huggins and Hodges had won a Nobel Prize in medicine and physiology in 1966 for their discovery.

Without the presence of testosterone, most prostate cancer cells shrivel up and die. But eventually they will find another growth factor to help them propagate and proliferate. These cancer cells have a mind of their own, the same desperate desire to survive and reproduce that I had. A formidable opponent.

Eunuchs – young boys in various cultures who have been castrated in order to make them into couriers and servants and guardians of women and high-pitched singers – never develop prostate cancer. They are immune because of their inability to produce testosterone in their castrated state. I on the other hand was facing the worst of all worlds—being a eunuch *and* having prostate cancer.

A new kind of castration anxiety. A literal castration terror. Sigmund Freud coined the term, castration anxiety, as a metaphor for the struggles every adult male and female, gay or straight, feels in an ongoing relationship—the struggles in being able to combine a sense of grounding with a genuine sharing of passions in a steadfast relationship. Many of us can have one or the other, but we can feel swallowed up in a relationship—we lose ourselves, we lose our solid sense of identity—when we try to establish both facets in a relationship. It is what's called the classic Madonna-whore complex, except it occurs just as readily for women as for men, just as readily for gays as for straights. Some of us turn to our partners for grounding and support and nurturing. Others of us turn to our partners for the relief of unbearable sexual urges. Often the twain never meet—or at least do not meet in the same partner. We turn to one partner for grounding and support and to another for the sharing of passions—a phenomenon we can observe in presidents of the United States, in governors of New York, a ubiquitous phenomenon.

Freud's choice of words was unfortunate. Being swallowed up, losing one's sense of self, being overwhelmed by the demands of a relationship: None of these are akin to castration, especially for women.

Let's deal with the real deal, not the metaphor. No metaphors using the notion of castration are allowed in the late twentieth and early twenty-first centuries. Huggins and Hodges with their Nobel Prize-winning research in 1944 made sure of that. Now prostate cancer and real castration go hand in hand.

The surgeon in Manhattan made that case stridently. After poking and prodding and prying around in the soft tissue around my anus (I was under general anesthesia), he later told me that castration was absolutely essential.

"Even though we haven't found any clear-cut cancer cells, it doesn't mean the cancer isn't there. All the literature indicates that the sooner you get castrated the better. Waiting will only lead to your dying sooner."

He handed me some journal articles from the *New England Journal of Medicine*, which I looked over halfheartedly. I got the gist: In one way or another I would be dying very, very soon—either a metaphorical death by a literal castration or a literal death via metastatic prostate cancer.

"You have two choices—a chemical castration using medication to shut down your hypothalamus and pituitary and by extension your testicles, or a surgical castration. I can arrange to do the surgical castration here at the hospital. Just say the word."

I was speechless.

Eventually, I simply said, "Let me get back to DC as soon as possible. I'll talk to Helen, I'll think it over, and I'll let you know. Don't schedule the surgical castration quite yet."

All I knew was that I was fucked. The classic Hobbesian choice: I will not be able to fuck if alive, or the prostate cancer gods are really fucking with life itself.

—⁓—

"I'm taking some time off from work," I told my colleagues at Georgetown University. "It could be a few days, a few weeks, I don't know how long it will be." They all seemed to be okay with it. I had told them about some "major complications" with my prostate cancer.

I gathered around my closest friends, along with Helen, and explained my dilemma: "It seems like surgical castration or chemical castration is inevitable—sooner rather than later according to everyone I've spoken to so far." We were sitting in my downstairs office at home, trying to troubleshoot. We all knew the trouble, but none of us had any bullets to shoot with.

Finally, in the midst of a despairing silence, one of my friends piped up, "You've gotten to this point by talking to the best minds in the medical business. You've never failed to get alternative viewpoints and recommendations. This is not a good time to drop that approach."

This idea broke the impasse. Speaking to someone, an expert, anyone, had to be better than sitting there in a helpless castration-panic mode.

I got on the horn trying to figure out how to reach Gerald Murphy, who along with his colleagues had developed the prostate-specific antigen, the PSA, a few years before in a lab in a hospital in Buffalo, New York. If anyone might know how to interpret the PSA of 2.1 and what to do about it, he would be the man.

It took me about forty minutes to track him down—remember, this was long before the Internet and search engines. Murphy, it turned out, moved from Buffalo to Atlanta and was now working at the Center for Disease Control (CDC). Amazingly, I was able to reach him on my first try.

My voice quivering, my speech pressured—with my cascading terror I barely had had any sleep for several days—I summarized my story and current predicament, with my rising PSA and a normal bone scan.

I heard giggling on the other end. Is this guy some imperious and insensitive jerk who thinks he is a gift from the gods to our lowly planet?

Boy, were my initial impressions wrong. I never had the pleasure of meeting Gerald Murphy in person before he passed away eleven years later from a heart attack while attending a conference in Israel, yet at that very moment, Murphy actually saved my life. He saved the basic fabric of my life—my work life, my family life, my marriage, my life as a man. He gave me a reprieve from castration, from the testicular guillotine.

"Listen, I'm only laughing because of the unnecessary panic in you and your doctors. Relax, go back to work. Go back to your office and help some people who truly need some help, unlike yourself. You're fine. You'll have a nice decent life. There is absolutely no need to panic.

"Here's the thing: The PSA is a relatively new test as you know, and practitioners have not figured out how to use it and interpret it. I've had a number of post-prostatectomy patients whom I've followed for several years with experimental PSAs, before the PSA became a commercially available screening test. Some patients have had their PSAs rise to 18 or 20 without any evidence of palpable or visible disease. Your PSA will probably rise slowly over the next few years. The PSA of 2.1, without much doubt, reflects some existing disease, but the disease load is small and inconsequential. In a few years when the cancer becomes more consequential, you can consider some interventions.

"And, who knows?" he reminded me. "We might have some more benign treatments than castration in a few years." I wanted to tell him I could barely imagine any treatment being less benign than castration.

Dr. Murphy assured me that I could safely buy more time. "It's foolish to treat a blood test, particularly a blood test whose implications are not as yet known. It's especially absurd to treat a blood test with a brutal assault on your testicles!"

My thoughts precisely. Gerald Murphy and John Maynard Keynes on the same wavelength. No one can predict the impact of new ideas and new inventions. Let me just stay alive to be able to see those new inventions and new interventions.

Murphy's calming and reassuring words ring loud and undiminished thirty years later, and they will remain so for the rest of my life.

—m—

One of the most gratifying parts of being a physician is the impact we can have on others when we least expect it. A simple suggestion, a throwaway comment, a brief insight—we might find out years later this comment made a major difference in a person's life. It is all in the timing and in the degree of distress and one's corresponding openness to a new perspective. My conversation with Gerald Murphy had all three elements. I was open to anything that provided a counterpoint to the terror-inducing agenda of castration.

Although I never spoke to Murphy again, even to thank him profusely, his comments have allowed me to ward off the persistent and insistent suggestions over the last twenty-five years to have my testicles removed. One academic oncologist a few years later had the hubris to tell me that emotionally I would be better off castrated.

Surprised that I had not already succumbed to a chemical or surgical castration for my long-term survival, he added, "With castration, at least you never have to worry about your potency, you never have to worry about getting it up. If you don't have any libido, you don't have to worry about performance. It makes thing less complicated."

Come again? The ultimate Orwellian doublespeak. How crucial is it to get a second or third or fourth opinion when you recognize how crazy some of my medical colleagues are? Not crazy in the conventional sense, but how distorted their views may be because of their backgrounds and their own traumas and their own personal crises and their own personal way of relating to the world. Helen had pointed out to me repeatedly in medical school that no sane person would voluntarily go to some of my classmates once these classmates became physicians. What do the comments from the oncologist above tell us about his romantic and sexual life, about his desires for intimacy, and about his desire to satisfy a partner as well as himself? Only later did I find out he was going through a messy divorce at the time.

When we encounter the Gerald Murphys of the world—maybe if I had gotten to meet him and know him, he would have turned out to be a crazy old coot himself—all we can do is savor the encounter, and hold onto it for dear life.

—⚏—

Over the years I have grown to love the PSA. Patients with breast cancer and other cancers would love to have a similar marker. The PSA is indeed specific to the prostate; its source is the prostate and only the prostate. When the prostate has been removed or obliterated by surgery or radiation, there should be no PSA circulating in our bloodstreams. It is a perfect marker for determining whether a recurrence has developed and how fast it is growing.

At the same time, the PSA has been a mixed blessing for men who still have their prostates. It has become a ubiquitous screening tool for determining whether a man might have prostate cancer to begin with. A PSA above 4.0 has been arbitrarily set as abnormal. Yet we see plenty of false positives—men who have a PSA well above 4.0 with no sign of malignant disease, and some false negatives— men who have a PSA below 4.0 who may be harboring a cancer.

And, if a cancer is found, using the new fiber-optic cystoscopies not available in 1984, we still do not know which ones will remain localized in situ cancers and which ones will become aggressive and metastatic.

Gerald Murphy was correct twenty-six years ago: We still do not know how to interpret the PSA, although we have a better understanding of its meaning after the prostate has been removed.

In the meantime I had *the* man, *the* expert on PSAs in my hip pocket, in my very being, reinforcing the idea that castration would not be imminent. Yet I knew that castration could be put off for only so long. How would I cope with this eventuality, especially after years of putting forth a special effort to regain my sexual energies and my sexual capacities, and love and romance?

It did not take a long time to find out.

CHAPTER 12

This Way for the Testicle Remover, Eunuchs and Gentlemen

"It is not so much a matter of playing a good hand well; it is much more a matter of how well we play a bad hand."
—Robert Louis Stevenson

I could now talk prostate cancer lingo with the best of them. My own hubris startled me. One cannot underestimate the impact of a death sentence or a castration sentence. Out of desperation can come a full personality change. Normally shy and retiring, I somehow found a way to take on an air of confidence in presenting crucial questions to busy experts.

My hubris had been helped along by positive reinforcement—read, Gerald Murphy. When faced with experts, I was able to seal over any discouragement and come across as a fellow expert who was simply picking their brain for a new insight or a new discovery. These contacts were often swift and to the point, unmemorable and mercifully brief perhaps for the physician, but extraordinarily memorable for me.

I may have been appealing to these experts' healthy narcissism and their healthy desire to share with the world their ideas and inventions and breakthroughs. I was also appealing to their altruistic bent, their desire to help a young colleague. They could relate and identify with me, and if they had any sadistic bent, it was not visible in this context.

In some cockeyed way these prostate cancer experts had wandered into a career that catered almost exclusively to septuagenarians and octogenarians. They were catering to the anuses and penises of alter-kockers—a term from Yiddish that is sometimes defined kindly as "old defecator." These physicians were probably overjoyed to encounter a youngish guy like me who did not reek of urine and feces, and who could take their insights and advice and run with these ideas, with the possibility, though improbable, for a long life ahead. Luck and skill and hubris—the very things I would need in short order.

—⁂—

The PSA continued to rise. By early 1992, three years after the initial early signs of a rising PSA, it was now up to 6.3, and I was getting a little more than nervous. Out of the blue, though—luck and serendipity are all-important in life—I got a call from my surgeon in New York City.

"Listen, two of my colleagues, researchers here, are beginning a study of monoclonal antibodies, to help in determining the whereabouts of prostate cancer in people like yourself with rising PSAs post-prostatectomy. You're a perfect candidate for this research—you have recurrent disease but we have no idea where to find it. Your bone scans have fortunately all been negative, showing no evidence of disease. So, this study can be a very useful diagnostic test. And who knows? Eventually we may be able to use monoclonal antibodies as a treatment to attack the remaining disease."

Sounded good to me. I was aware of the promise of monoclonal antibodies, a promise not truly realized at least partially until twenty years later. The premise was a reasonable one: Let's find a specific antigen or protein from prostate cancer that can stimulate antibodies. Then let's attach chemicals or radiation or viruses or bacteria to these antibodies that will go specifically to the cancer cells and kill them—without any collateral damage of killing healthy cells. Highly targeted chemotherapy or radiotherapy or pathogen therapy. In my case, though, they were only looking to see where the antibodies might be heading, without the antibodies having any killer capabilities.

I hopped up to New York and the researchers injected me with radio-florescent prostate antibodies with the hope that they would gravitate to the elusive cancer cells. Afterwards, the younger of the two researchers sat down with me after lunch. "Our study shows significant cancer cells in multiple lymph nodes along your abdominal aorta and along the carotid artery in your neck. You appear to have a great deal of disease."

Subsequent CT scans and MRIs of these areas did not confirm any unusual lymph nodes. All the nodes along my aorta and carotid artery were small and unobtrusive, under one centimeter in width and length.

"We've arranged for a vascular surgeon here at the hospital to dissect your carotid artery this afternoon. A surgical suite is ready and waiting. We want to do this procedure as soon as possible. Despite the CTs and MRIs, we think you have real and genuine, though microscopic, disease, and we want to confirm the findings of the radio-florescent antibodies."

Okay, you are scaring the shit out of me. These two researchers were convincing me it was essential to see where my rising PSA was coming from, yet I knew that dissecting a carotid artery was not without risk.

I quickly called my internist in Washington, DC. To my surprise, I was able to reach him directly, and I succinctly told him the story. He listened quietly, and after a brief moment of silence, he said, through seemingly clenched teeth—this is a guy I had never heard curse—"Get the fuck out of there before they kill you."

I needed this swift and sober assessment. Anxious to please, I got caught up in the agenda of the researchers. Yes, boxers box, surgeons cut, and researchers do research. Like hedgehogs they know one thing very, very well. But they may not have the multiple interests and skills and sensitivities of the fox. My own survival was now diverging from the researchers' desire to flourish in their careers.

I hightailed out of there in a flash.

In the twenty-three years since then, there have been no sightings of cancer cells anywhere near my aorta and carotid arteries.

—✲—

Before rushing out of Manhattan, though, I followed through on a vow I made before the trip to use the time there as effectively as possible. I made an appointment with the purported king of prostate oncology at Sloan-Kettering Cancer Center, with the hope of just picking his brain and seeing what alternatives there were to castration.

Two hours after the designated appointment time, he raced into the examining room. "I already know a lot about your case," he noted, much to my surprise. He had just had dinner with the two researchers the night before. "The best and most prudent course for you is immediate castration. There really are no other alternatives. There are some new interesting medications in the pipeline to induce a chemical castration. A new drug Casadex is coming out of England for that purpose."

I was only half listening. Gerald Murphy's words were swirling in the other half of my ears and brain.

In almost a throwaway line, he remarked, "There is an oncologist in Vancouver, British Columbia, who is doing some interesting work with an intermittent androgen blockade, an intermittent chemical castration. But you're not a suitable candidate for that approach. Your cancer is too advanced and too aggressive, your PSA has risen too high and too rapidly, and now there is evidence of spread of the disease to the lymph nodes along your aorta and carotids. I really think you should have a surgical castration, to rid yourself completely and permanently of all testosterone."

Fortunately Gerald Murphy was still swirling in my head. And who was this guy in Vancouver?

—⁓—

Permanent surgical castration eventually will go the way of leeches and other bizarre and foolhardy medical interventions. But bucking the medical establishment when it has a particular approach, a virtual ideology for understanding or treating a medical condition, is nearly impossible. The medical establishment may be wrong but it is never in doubt. Those same sadistic medical students who loved doing invasive procedures in the third year of medical school also seem to have the cockiness years later to establish the medical ideologies that control treatment protocols. One needs an iconoclast, someone who is thinking differently yet coherently, to buck the tides.

Nicholas Bruchovsky was just that iconoclast. As soon as I arrived home from New York City, I called him in Vancouver. An American-trained oncologist, Nick had been doing his research in cancer endocrinology in relative obscurity in the Canadian health care system, the equivalent of Siberia. He was delighted to explain his research to me over the phone, happy that someone was listening.

"More is not always more, more is not always better," he pointed out. Less is sometimes more, according to what I now call the "wisdom of Nick." "If castration works to eliminate testosterone as a growth factor for prostate cancers, then Western doctors tend to keep that intervention going indefinitely. But castration only works effectively for a matter of months or at most a few years. Eventually with testosterone gone, the cancer cells find a way to establish some other protein or hormone as a growth factor or growth stimulus. Huggins and Hodges realized that less might be better even in the 1940s. But everyone seemed to ignore that message."

Yeah, bombs away. If something works, simply bombard the organism with more and more of that potent intervention. Heap it on, pile it up. Chemotherapy? Let's do mega-chemotherapy, even if it means destroying the bone marrow and killing the patient. At least we've killed the cancer.

Nick seemed to get it: Permanent castration was not the equivalent of, say, the lancing of a skin lesion. Most of the rest of the medical establishment: No lumpectomies allowed, instead let's remove everything—the breasts and the vaginas and the penises and, above all, the testicles.

"You're an ideal candidate for this approach. You have PSA-only recurrent prostate cancer. There are no signs of any visible recurrence. And the evidence is that this intermittent chemical castration, this intermittent androgen blockade does no worse than a permanent blockade. And there is a very good chance it might do better in the long run than a permanent blockade. And the quality of your life . . ."

Say no more, Nick. Rarely is one approach *infinitely* better in its side effects than another approach. Let's see: Zero sexual life for the rest of my life versus a sexual capacity for as much as two-thirds of the rest of my life. My penis put away for life or my penis imprisoned for eight-month sentences every two years or so.

Plus, we would be having fun fooling the cancer cells. They were fucking with me, and we would be fucking with them. Nick and I as co-conspirators: We'll give those fucking cells all the testosterone they want and need in order to survive and thrive; then we'll take away the testosterone and they'll quiver and shrivel. Then, just when they are about to hunt around for some other substance to fuel their growth, we'll hit them with a heavy dose of testosterone again. They'll then stop looking for some other stimulus for their growth.

My interests and the interests of the cancer cells were actually in line: When they were shriveling, my testicles were likewise fizzling and my penis drooping. When they were blooming, my testicles were expanding and my penis was poised and proud.

A new kind of zero-sum game. A new kind of equilibrium, a matching of wits. You guys will eventually kill me but not without a fight. And both of us will survive, not necessarily happily all of the time, but we'll both have what we want and need a good part of the time. Sometimes it will be win-win; then it will be lose-lose.

In some ways I might have had a competitive advantage. Even in the midst of castration, I had something remarkable to look forward to—a return to arousal and excitement and bliss. I had a will to live that would match the cancer cells' will to live. Perhaps this was the message of Wilhelm Reich: A man without a sex drive, a man without orgasms, a man without romance, a man without dreams of sexual conquests, a man without a capacity to fully respond to his partner— that man may lose his will to live. As his testicles shriveled, so would he. Other forms of cancer as well as diabetes, heart disease, drug and alcohol problems, depression and suicidality—all of these maladies could kill him.

So, bring on that orgone box, bring back those orgasms, bring back that male rapaciousness. I was still alive and kicking. I would be buying some time in this equilibrium with my cancer, hoping for some new breakthroughs and inventions in treating the cancer, and looking for some greater competitive advantage while in my current steady state.

Helen was more than comfortable with this plan and with the wisdom of Nick. We would work together to find a way to make this temporary castration manageable. We had time to figure it out, to build more romance into our lives—the PSA had not reached a level yet for me to start the chemical castration, but that was coming soon, coming soon to a theater near me.

Yes, cool moss. When facing fierce fiery coals, think "cool moss," and walk in a directed and purposeful way, and keep your eyes on the desired outcome without a sense of desperation and panic. Above all do not run; do not trip and fall. Keep your eyes on the prize of life itself and the prize of a soon-to-be staggered sexual vitality.

CHAPTER 13

Youth is Wasted on the Young

"If youth knew; if age could."

—Estienne

"Only a moment; a moment of strength, of romance, of glamour—of youth! . . . A flick of sunshine upon a strange shore, the time to remember, the time for a sigh, and—good-bye!—Night—Good-bye . . . !"

—Joseph Conrad, *Youth*

". . . when thou art old and rich, Thou hast neither heat, affection, limb, nor beauty
To make thy riches pleasant."

—William Shakespeare, *Measure for Measure*

I found the fountain of youth. Juan Ponce de Leon, eat your heart out—you were five hundred years too late. This fountain of youth is not in Florida, Juan, nor is it anything you ever could have wished for. Be careful what you wish for, old Ponce. There is no free lunch. With the fountain of youth come hardships; with dreams come discomforts.

At age sixty-six I may look as much as ten to fifteen years younger than my age. I have a full head of hair with virtually no gray hair. I barely have any wrinkles. Despite a bit of plumpness in the midsection, I do not look all that different than when I was in my twenties or thirties. I still play basketball regularly, and I still jump as high as I could forty-five years ago—not very high. Some of these youthful twists may be tied in with my genes, but most of these twists come from this fountain of youth.

I am also starting my tenth adolescence—nine of them since age forty-four, over a twenty-two year period. *Groundhog Day* personified. Who the hell is writing this screenplay, this trajectory of a crazy life? The gods have set it up so that in one of these puberties I will eventually get it right.

In my first experience of adolescence, puberty started at twelve, in 1960. It was a good enough set of teenage years, not necessarily filled with the teen angst that many people describe. I was adept in school, played sports, had good friends, and hung out with my fellow high schoolers at the local ice cream shop. A few of us would head up to the New York border where the drinking age was eighteen instead of Connecticut's twenty-one. We hung out at a bar in Port Chester (a town we called Sin City) that must have paid off the police. We never showed IDs and were able to drink at sixteen. I did not have high alcohol tolerance so I had a few close calls with intoxication and made a fool of myself more than once, but no big deal.

I never got laid in junior high or high school. I was too shy; I hadn't developed any good pickup lines; I fumbled around when it came to girls.

But there was no need to replay this phase of my life, especially nine more times. Especially since replaying it meant going through childhood again. See, to reach puberty nine more times, you have no choice but to go back to prepuberty nine more times.

Prepuberty sucks. You lose the hair on your chest. Your skin becomes soft and smooth. You lose your muscle mass. You become, once again, a ninety-eight-pound weakling. If you are a baseball pitcher, you lose at least twenty miles per hour on your fastball. If you are a golfer, your two-hundred-yard tee shots become seventy-five-yard dribblers. If you are a tennis player, you begin to rely on drop shots. Ah, the fountain of youth.

It is the exact opposite of the steroid age in sports. Those of us with metastatic prostate cancer have had our 'droids taken away. The most flattering comment for real athletes: He is a man among boys. No, I am a boy among men.

Admittedly, with the coming of these past nine puberties and adolescences, I do get laid right away. No fumbling around, no need for pickup lines, no concerns about shyness. Almost a biblical kind of adolescence: You reach puberty, you are married at the start of this adolescence, and you can start getting laid as soon as you reach puberty. No arranged marriage—but you do need a willing partner who is somehow willing to go through her partner's nine trips through prepuberty. But no need for masturbation, no need for onanism when you reread this adolescence. Biblical strictures from twenty-seven hundred years ago make sense in this one and only context.

A fluorescent adolescence—a flowering now nine extra times with the re-advent of testosterone, with the re-advent of puberty. I still have not gotten prepuberty and puberty right despite my ten tries. I hope to keep going, though, through an eleventh, a twelfth . . . Maybe I'll get it right the next time. Hope springs eternal. A pubertal spring brings hope.

—⚏—

By November 1992, my PSA had risen to 9.9. It was time to act. I quickly headed to Vancouver to meet with Nicholas Bruchovsky. Another Gerald-Murphy-like moment, but this time I actually met the man, the expert. Not unlike Gerald Murphy, he renewed my faith in man, in physicians, in myself. Sure, Nick had self-interest at heart just like the rest of us, but his compassion and genuine interest in me and my predicament came through immediately. He could relate fully to my desire to protect my testicles and avoid any permanent castration. And he had a plan.

We started on two drugs not typically used in the United States—first a tiny dose of diethylstilbesterol, or DES, the notorious fertility drug that was used in the 1940s. It had allowed women to get pregnant and have babies, but no one knew at the time that it would have horrific effects on the offspring and on future generations—not unlike radiation. These DES babies eventually developed vaginal cancers and infertility in adulthood.

Yet one person's poison is another person's salvation. No need for me to worry about vaginal cancer or infertility; I already had my own pelvic cancer and infertility.

The second drug was cyproterone acetate, developed as a steroidal anti-androgen by a German pharmaceutical company but not available in the United States. The company had gotten a rapid routine approval for the drug in Canada and Europe but encountered a more cumbersome and intimidating approval process in the United States. The hell with it, they decided—and men in the US have therefore been denied a reasonable and well-tolerated medication over the past thirty years.

After three or four weeks, we replaced the DES with an injectable medication called goserelin (Zoladex) that blocks the release of gonadotrophin in the hypothalamus and pituitary and in turn blocks the production of testosterone in the testicles. In Canada it was do-it-yourself. One of Nick's colleagues had me watch a video to learn how to inject the Zolodex subcutaneously, just under the skin, into my abdomen on a monthly—eventually every three-month—basis. No financial waste in the Canadian system, no need to go to the doctor for a simple injection.

"At some point the cyproterone acetate will not work quite as well as it does now. The cancer will develop some resistance to its effects," Nick noted. "But we have a bunch of nonsteroidal anti-androgens waiting in the wings—flutamide and nilutamide and a new one called bicalutamide." The same drug the Sloan-Kettering guy had touted a year or two earlier.

"We'll use these drugs sequentially over the years, and you should be able to get some good mileage out of each of these medications."

Although we were talking about castration—making my big cojones into smaller and smaller cojones—Nick's conversational style was reassuring and gave me the sense that this literal emasculation would be manageable, especially since it was temporary and reversible.

This gentle and kindly prince of a man I began to picture, rightly or wrongly, as a patrician White Russian who seemed still genuinely confused and troubled by the Russian Revolution seventy-five years earlier. Who are these guys, Marx and Lenin and Trotsky? Where did they come from? Why are they and their ideas screwing up a stable monarchy and a stable country? Couldn't we have gone the way of Britain, limiting the power of the kings and queens while creating a new power structure, without some violent revolution? Okay, so we won't call Catherine "great" anymore. And then he found himself practicing medicine in Canada, in a socialist medical care system. Was he simply trying to understand and master the events of 1917?

But money did not appear to be a motivating force. He just wanted to get the word out about the wisdom of this intermittent androgen blockade, about less being more, or less at least being the same and no worse than more. All this from the backwaters of Vancouver, from where chauvinist Americans dismiss any new notions and findings.

And Nick implicitly wanted to ask the right questions of his patients who had metastatic prostate cancer. How important is it for you to continue to be a sexual being? How awful will it be for you to be permanently asexual? How much pride and dignity will you lose with a permanent castration? In essence, is sex important to you?

Some men and women would reluctantly acknowledge that sex is not important to them. Take out those damn testicles, take out those damn ovaries, take out all those damn hormones produced by those testicles and ovaries. Who needs them? We all have different hopes and dreams, different priorities, different agendas, different yearnings and longings, different fears and anxieties.

Some patients and their physicians may not be able to live with the ambiguity and uncertainty of a nonpermanent castration. Let's go with the accepted protocol. Let's not ask too many questions. Let's not try anything new and offbeat. Just choose: your testicles or your life.

With Nick I would not have to choose and face this Hobbesian choice. I could have my cake and eat it too; I could have my life and beat it too. Keep my nutsack—temporarily out of commission—and keep my life. All my efforts to recover from the ravages of prostate cancer treatments would not be in vain. The hyperbaric oxygen, the acupuncture, the return of erections and sexual revelry—no, all was not lost.

—⁂—

Within twelve days after initiating the chemical castration in December 1992, my PSA dropped from 9.9 to 2.7. Seven months later the PSA was down to undetectable levels, less than 0.06. In the face of castration I was at least getting remarkable results. The prostate cancer was temporarily in retreat.

I was also in retreat—a castrated retreat. No sex life, no fantasy life, no double entendres. Yes, I have found the fountain of youth. I am young after my time. I am not aging in the same way as my peers, many of whom are old before their time. And my youth is not wasted while being young—I have found ways to waste my youth while growing old.

Yet I do *not* grow old . . . I do *not* grow old, I shall *not* wear my trousers rolled. This fountain of youth, though, is a piece of crap, a piece of trash, not all that it is cracked up to be. Better to age and die in the usual and customary ways. This fountain of youth—F'get about it.

Yes, I have heard the mermaids sing, each to each. Yet I can only hope they will return to sing to me. They are not singing to me now. I have indeed seen the moment of my greatness flicker. A new kind of metaphorical death. How do I cope? What does this all mean? What is the meaning of life, the meaning of death, the meaning of love and sex? How do I cope even with a temporary castration?

Can I maintain a healthy mind in the face of castration? And can healthy mind and castration be used in the same sentence?

CHAPTER 14

Redemption, of Sorts

There lives more faith in honest doubt,
Believe me, than in half the creeds.
                              —Alfred, Lord Tennyson

I am for religion against religions.
                              —Victor Hugo, *Les Miserables*

Faith is to believe what we do not see; and the reward of this
faith is to see what we believe.
                              —St. Augustine

I believe in the sun even when it is not shining.
I believe in love even when not feeling it.
I believe in God even when God appears to be silent.
            —Inscription on a cellar wall in Cologne in 1943

I can believe anything, provided it is incredible.
            —Oscar Wilde, *The Picture of Dorian Gray*

Imagine the kind of punitive gods we can create in thinking about
prostate cancer. If HIV became a punitive symbol in the late
twentieth century for the profligate sexuality of the 1960s, imagine

the field day we can have with prostate cancer, especially when it hits young men like myself.

Can the gods create any better scourge against human sexuality? Let's see what we sadistic fuckers up in the heavens can do to those cocksure heathens down below. Let's create erectile dysfunction and impotence and loss of jism and loss of fertility and loss of libido all in one fell swoop. Let's create a disease that will force the caregivers to lance and slash pelvises, then burn and radiate the base of penises. Then for good measure we'll see if the caregivers might realize—hey, we'll give a couple of scientists the Nobel Prize for discovering this intervention—that cutting off a guy's balls might give the guy a few more years to live. Surgical hell, radiation hell, castration hell. Even Dante could not have imagined these circles of hell.

Nothing cures societal licentiousness and salaciousness like prostate cancer. Better than HIV disease. A right-winger's wet dream, a religious zealot's wet dream. No wanton sex, no pregnancies—no sleeping around and no creation of single-parent families and no unwanted children and no potential abortions. No male homosexuality—or male heterosexuality, for that matter. No male sexual assaults or rapes. Prostate cancer for every adult male, and all our social ills are solved.

I do not want any part of these social cures and these gods. No need for guilt-inducing gods, no need for terrorizing gods, no need for vengeful gods—gods that, with society's crazy projections, are punishing people because of, say, the supposed depravity of an era, of a nation, of a particular ethnic group, of a particular sexual orientation.

Studies show that highly religious people too often give up on treatment for a potentially deadly condition. No point in trying to regain one's health: I have screwed up; I have sinned; I have gotten what I deserve. My fate is sealed. All I can do is accept the punishment I deserve. A helplessness and hopelessness that take on a life of their own.

Yet I wanted and needed gods—gods that were comforting and reassuring. I have had enough terror with my castration anxiety. Enough. As the atheist and physicist Freeman Dyson has pointed out, most atheists do not understand and appreciate the "anguish" of religious believers—an anguish that cannot help but induce some kind of religious belief. I was a walking embodiment of this anguish.

History is filled with tales of presumably sane people undergoing religious conversions in the face of life-threatening illnesses. The writer Walker Percy converted to Catholicism after his confrontation with tuberculosis as a young man. The singer-songwriter Cat Stevens, who had a remarkable run of creativity in his teens and early twenties, converted to Islam after almost drowning, which followed shortly on the heels of a diagnosis of tuberculosis. Leo Tolstoy went through a major religious phase in his later years as he faced his fragility and mortality. There may be something wrong with a picture of any sentient human being facing his fragility and death without some kind of change in perspective, without some kind of attitude adjustment, without some kind of spiritual awakening, whatever that notion means.

Human beings have been around for approximately 150,000 years, of which most of these millennia have been filled with human aggressiveness and impulsivity and violence. Religions were essential in binding us together as tight-knit groups, to face challenges and battles—wars to the death—with other equally tight-knit religious groups.

But I was not in a battle with any human enemy. I was locked in battle with prostate cancer and the forces that were gradually taking more and more of my pelvic functioning away from me.

In the ancient religions of our hunter-gatherer ancestors, long before humans became settled ten thousand years ago (with the stabilization of the earth's climate), people felt they were communicating with the supernatural world through dreams and trances. Through these séances and hypnotic reveries, they asked their gods for practical help in their survival—good hunting and good weather, successful healing and health, triumphant outcomes in battles and wars.

Trances appear to have been a central feature of any of the ancient religions that predated the major monotheistic religions. As Nicholas Wade notes in *The Faith Instinct*, "In a survey of almost five hundred small-scale societies, the anthropologist Erika Bourguignon found that 90 percent had rites in which regular trance states occurred, data for the other 10 percent being insufficient to know whether or not this was the case."

In contrast, the modern religions, developing in settled societies with the advent of agriculture and the domestication of animals and other food sources, have produced a priestly class of rabbis and imams and priests and ministers that direct people toward what happens *after* we die, to the after-death, to the afterlife. These modern monotheistic religions have been essential in organizing and controlling a larger and more settled society—to keep people in line via threats of what can happen in the afterlife if they do not follow the religion's and society's tenets.

It may not be too simplistic to say that the co-religionists in an ancient hunting and gathering society attempted to achieve salvation and survival in the real world, whereas the followers of modern religions have been more focused on survival and salvation in the illusory afterlife.

No surprise then that my focus was much more in line with the religions of the ancient world. Mesmer continued to be my guide—mesmerism and the trance, as defined by Gilbert Rouget as a "transcendence of one's normal self, as a liberation resulting from the intensification of a mental or physical disposition, in short, as an exaltation . . . of the self." I harked back to the root for "enthusiasm," the Greek word *enthousiasmos* meaning "being possessed by a god."

I will speak in tongues; I will sing and dance the night away; I will muster heavenly amounts of enthusiasm; I will become possessed by the gods. A cult of one, a religion of one.

Perhaps I will pray to the old Greek and Roman gods of fertility and love and sexuality, Eros and Cupid. I desperately and enthusiastically needed them—to sustain my sexuality, to maintain my capacity for love, to regain my fertility. Who the hell pushed them out of favor?

Who the hell and what the hell determines for us what kind of gods we believe in and pray to? It seems all predetermined simply by the family we happen to be born into. If we are born into a Muslim family, we become Muslim; Christian family, then a Christian; Jewish, Hindu, Buddhist, you name it. If we are born into an atheistic family, we will probably become atheists ourselves. We may assert some modest control by leaving certain sects and joining other sects within that same religion. If we marry into another religion, we may feel some pressure to leave our religion and join the one of our spouse. But our family of origin asserts enormous control. At the height of our suggestibility and hypnotizability, we get inculcated with a belief system that is almost impossible to shake. Training in the religion of our fathers and mothers, in the religion of our grandfathers and grandmothers, takes hold of us and will not let go.

Yet the notion of a god or gods is merely a projection, a Rohrschach card that can be interpreted in myriad ways—with no right or wrong answer—an inkblot that represents our own projections and assumptions and experiences and schooling, along with all our hopes and fears and yearnings.

Can we liberate ourselves from the god or gods of our fathers, the god or gods of our mothers? Literally, no. Transference rules us and controls us. Transference: the ubiquitous process by which we create internal representations of current people in our lives—be it spouses, lovers, bosses, teachers, coaches, clergymen—based on past important people in our childhoods, usually parents and siblings.

Our view of God is mostly a transference phenomenon, as the psychoanalyst Ana-Maria Rizzuto has pointed out. Our internal representation of god or the gods is remarkably congruent with our internal representation of our parents or other crucial parenting figures. In case after case she describes men and women whose view of God is virtually the same as the way they view their parents. If they grew up with a punitive parent, their god is punitive. If they grew up with parents who were dismissive and abandoning, their god is dismissive and aloof.

Atheists are not immune from this transference phenomenon. If they have grown up with grotesquely abusive parents, they may reject these parents and may reject all gods. If they feel poorly understood by a parent or parents, they cannot imagine a god or gods that can accept them and understand them.

Here is an example from Rizzuto's work—a comparison of one man's statements about God and statements about his father:

I have never experienced closeness to God.	I was never close to my father.
If I am in distress, I do not resort to God, because I have no belief in God.	I do not ask anything from my father.
I do not formally pray, but I may toss a coin in a fountain and make a wish or think in a hopeful way because it makes me feel good.	I don't talk to my father.

We human beings cannot win. Whether we like it or not, we are products of our experiences, products of our childhoods, products of our heightened hypnotizability during that childhood.

Our illusions are based on the reality of our lives. Our God delusion is no more an illusion than militant modern atheism is an illusion. Rizzuto again: "To ask a man to renounce a god he believes in may be as cruel and as meaningless as wrenching a child from his teddy bear so that he can grow up . . . Asking a mature, functioning individual to renounce his God would be like asking Freud to renounce his own creation, psychoanalysis, and the 'illusory' promise of what scientific knowledge can do . . . Men cannot be without illusions. The type of illusion we select—science, religion, or something else—reveals our personal history . . ." Likewise, to ask a man to renounce atheism may be just as cruel and as meaningless as . . .

Time for me now to select my own specific illusions, my own specific gods. The wonderful thing about adulthood is that we can personally select our own friends, our partners, our mentors—and our own gods. As kids we are a captive audience, stuck with the family, gods, illusions, and religion we are born into.

Those of us who have had the good fortune of growing up with nonpunitive parents also have the enhanced good fortune of being able to create a loving and comforting and encouraging set of gods inside our heads. A well-nurtured childhood can be a gift that keeps on giving. In contrast, adults raised in childhood by punitive parents have no such luck. The gods inside their heads only make them crazier and more neurotic, and they often thrust their punitive gods on the rest of us.

So, I wanted and needed gods that could support me through my grief. In 1984, with the initial diagnosis of prostate cancer and the subsequent surgery, mourning had dawned; mourning had broken. Shock and bargaining and anger and despair—all the steps any of us go through in grappling with grief and loss—were a staple of my life.

But with whom do I bargain? I have bargained with friends and colleagues and storekeepers and car dealers over material goods, but not so effectively over life and death stuff.

And at whom should I express my absolute outrage over my plight? No point in displacing my anger toward Helen or my friends or my doctors. My rage had to be directed somewhere, toward someone or something—no point in squashing it or suppressing it. If we did not have the "God of our fathers" to whom to express our ire, we would have to invent some other gods. Fuck it, if Job can express his rage at God, so can I express my rage at any gods of my choosing.

I will also take Pascal's "wager" one step further. Blaise Pascal was a seventeenth-century mathematician who laid the theoretical foundations for measuring risk and probability. In his book, *Pensees*, he included a fragment asking, "God is, or he is not. Which way should we incline? Reason cannot answer." Only an illusory reason can answer.

The only way to choose in this coin flip between a bet that God exists and a bet that there is no God, is by deciding whether an outcome in which God exists is preferable. For Pascal the choice was a no-brainer. A belief in God promised salvation in the after-death.

Again, I wanted something more—salvation in the here and now. I did not give a shit about the afterlife, the after-death. If there was a 50 percent chance that a god or gods existed, then why not believe in these gods? If one believes in these gods, then why not accept, say, the 50 percent chance that these gods are comforting and encouraging and reassuring, not punitive? So, if we use Pascal's crazy fifty-fifty logic, there is a 25 percent chance that a caring and nurturing god or set of gods exists. One can create a whole new theology based on these simplistic statistical probabilities.

But I would allow none of the following bullshit in my spiritual life, in my religion—that "everything happens for a reason." I got prostate cancer for a "reason." I have been "chosen" for prostate cancer. I would not allow my silly illusory gods to become a source of militancy and a source of a sense of superiority.

The Jews got a lot of mileage out of the notion of being the "chosen people." A nice idea: We are special, we have been selected from all the tribes and nations of the world for special attention. Even if the Jews were ultimately selected for pogroms and extermination, they were able to put a positive spin on it. "Thank you, God, for choosing us to be Your victims and for making sure that our fellow man chooses us as his victim too." All said without a trace of irony.

But being a victim is a hell of a lot better than being ignored. Feeling "chosen" may have allowed the Jews to survive as a group, as a religion, as a nationality for centuries, whereas other ethnic groups may have disappeared.

In showering all this special attention on the chosen Jews, God received enormous attention in return. The more horrors this God handed out, the more religious many Jews became. Flog me more—I love it. Punish me, hurt me—I love my sadistic God.

Others found a way—much as I was doing—to find startling positives about God in the midst of horrors. They asked not "Where is God?" but instead "Where is man?" Man is an abomination; whereas God is great and beautiful. Man sucks, but God can do no wrong.

Admittedly, positive things come out of horrors. The Holocaust literature has been my friend, my companion since 1984, since the diagnosis of my prostate cancer. Yeah, I had prostate cancer to deal with, but at least I did not have to contend with the Nazis.

My favorite and arguably the best book on the Holocaust is *This Way for the Gas, Ladies and Gentlemen,* by Tadeusz Borowski, a non-Jew who survived the concentration camps. Here is an exchange in his title story—an exchange that reflects my own sense of priorities:

> . . . Directly beneath me, in the bottom bunk, lies a rabbi. He has covered his head with a piece of rag torn off a blanket and reads from a Hebrew prayer book (there is no shortage of this type of literature at the camp), wailing loudly, monotonously.
>
> "Can't somebody shut him up? He's been raving as if he'd caught God himself by the feet."

"I don't feel like moving. Let him rave. They'll take him to the oven that much sooner."

"Religion is the opium of the people," Henri, who is a Communist and a *rentier,* says sententiously. "If they didn't believe in God and eternal life, they'd have smashed the crematoria long ago."

"Why haven't you done it then?"

So, my gods are gods of action. One can get too much of prayer and meditation, too much also of passive Marxist determinism. We can engage in excesses of most anything. As Jacqueline Bouvier Kennedy Onassis is purported to have said in childhood, "Not lobster again tonight, Mother!" Chinese Daoists tell us that too much joy leads to heart disease.

A new vow began to evolve for me in the mid- and late 1980s, in the months and years just after surgery and radiation: I will make every effort to find a balance, to avoid excesses, to be conscious of the yin and the yang. I will be aware of potential errors of commission as well as potential errors of omission. I will be aware of the benefits, at times, of action and the benefits of inaction. I will find a balance that includes plenty of joy in the midst of grief. Some lobster, and yet not too much lobster.

Some people find their gods, their spiritual selves at the beach, at the ocean or sea with its endless horizons. I, though, wanted the solitude and privacy of a mountaintop—perhaps my own Mount Sinai. So, within months of the initial diagnosis, within months of surgery and radiation, I started heading up to the Shenandoah mountains— admittedly more like tall hills—ninety minutes from Washington, DC.

I found a mountain path just off Skyline Drive. It took only thirty minutes to climb to the top; and at the top I found an outcropping of rock fifty yards away from the trail that was at least fifteen or twenty feet higher than the elevation of the trail. It was an ideal spot for me to sit or stand or lie down as I talked to my gods, and it offered a swell view of the Shenandoah valley and river three thousand feet below and to the west.

My spot was far enough from the beaten track to allow me to rage against the gods, to cry uncontrollably whenever I wished, without being carted off by some worried hiker to the closest Virginia state mental hospital. Going up there monthly or bimonthly on a weekday, I rarely, if ever, encountered other hikers. My spot was always available—there were no other angry Job-like criers in this wilderness.

On my third visit, as I was meditating and talking to my gods, I noticed a small plaque nailed into the southern end of the rock outcropping. This metal plaque from the US Geological Survey noted that this very spot from which I was reaching out to the gods was the highest point in the Appalachians south of the Adirondacks. Had I randomly happened upon the Appalachian redneck equivalent of Mount Sinai? It even had its own insignia and polestar.

This modest find, this simple plaque, opened up the floodgates. All I could do was wail and rail. As much as I love rock 'n roll, wailin' and railin' is sometimes essential. These gods of my own creation, these illusions—not necessarily the God of my ancestors—accepted and tolerated all of my cries, my wails and rails. No back talk, no railing back at me, no punitive response. No, these gods of my own creation came through with comfort and encouragement—they were yes-gods. "Keep on doing what you're doing," was their implicit message.

No burning bush in this wilderness, no tablets filled with moral strictures for me to bring down from the mountain, no audible voices or palpable presence from these gods. That kind of god would have scared the shit out of me. No psychosis or temporal lobe epilepsy for me, thank you very much. I had enough problems.

These gods were veritable pussycats, quiet and unassuming. And I embraced these gods with unmitigated enthusiasm and hypnotic joy. In my own way I became possessed by these gods. On the mountaintop I was able to strengthen my hypnotic trance, to keep my eye on my goals, maintain hope, keep my focus, gain the energies necessary to achieve my seemingly impossible objectives. Yes, I will do everything humanly in my power to preserve my life and to preserve my sexual life. These gods of my creation will give me the courage, hubris even, to call the most significant people in any of the relevant scientific fields, to do everything I can to figure out the best course of action.

My world enlarged, and the Alps and the Rockies beckoned. Under the guise of these spiritual rounds, Helen and I, with our two daughters, headed off every few years—whenever we could put together enough money—to a tiny village in the Alps, accessible only by narrow-gauge railway. No cars, no pollution—the air was pristine. Several times during each of these trips, I went off for an afternoon by myself to a secluded mountain spot where I communed with my gods.

One afternoon after my communion with my gods, in the summer of 1992 when my PSA had begun to rise scarily, I met Helen and our daughters for a walk down to the village. At one point we took a short side trail that gave us a dazzling view of the glaciers and mountains above and the cliffs and valley below. There at the end of the trail, at the edge of the cliffs, stood almost as an apparition a family of four—a husband and wife and two daughters about the same age as ours. The man gestured to us, and his hardy "hello" told us they were Americans.

"Isn't this spot amazing?" he veritably shouted to us. Surprised to see anyone, let alone Americans, at this unusual spot, we quickly exchanged pleasantries. "We're from New York; I'm an oncologist in Manhattan. What brings you to this magical place?"

Helen and his wife began to talk separately, and all four kids broke off as well. The eight of us, now in three separate groups, started walking down the mountain. "To tell you the truth, we're here partly because of my prostate cancer. I head up into the mountains to, in a sense, meditate about my predicament and what to do about it." I did not normally tell strangers about my prostate cancer, but, hey, this guy had announced from the get-go he was an oncologist.

His ears perked up. "Did you know we're having more and more success using chemotherapy agents to treat prostate cancer? When the disease load is low, as in your case, we can intervene quite successfully. We've effectively treated guys with metastatic prostate cancer, guys who may have been on the brink of death months earlier."

Here I was on the edge of facing castration, with my PSA rising. Hope had taken a leap off the cliffs whether I was communing with my gods or not. And here came a mysterious stranger to announce that there was hope, that I might be able to resurrect myself, that there was such a thing as salvation in the here and now, not necessarily in the afterlife.

Although I did not follow through with any chemotherapy at that time—too little was known in the 1990s about how it might work in a slow-growing cancer like prostate cancer, and the effects of chemo may have been even more toxic than castration—I tucked away the information and let the sense of hope sweep over me. The salamander was going to resurrect his tail; the salamander was going to keep his third leg going even in the face of castration. I would continue to take action—meditation and wishful thinking had their place but action was crucial as well.

This disease would probably kill me, but not before I gave it a good ride, I thought. This cancer could possibly become a chronic long-lasting disease, not an immediate stone-cold killer.

CHAPTER 15

Psychotherapy for the Psychiatrist with Serious Castration Anxiety

"Desperate diseases require desperate remedies."

English Proverb

"He who has health has hope, and he who has hope has everything."

Arabian Proverb

"The mind is its own place, and in itself
Can make a heaven of hell, a hell of heaven."

John Milton, *Paradise Lost*

It takes a village to deal with and manage prostate cancer—an ethereal village in the heavens along with a palpable earthly village. Psychotherapy was and is a critical part of my earthly village.

We human beings have an optimism bias. People who are depressed and pessimistic have the most accurate handle on reality. They are acknowledging, instead of denying, the ubiquity of disease and trauma and death. The rest of us—with our often unfounded optimism and hopefulness—are in a state of denial and delusion. We are deliberately oblivious to life's afflictions. We assiduously avoid the nightside of life.

One of the ultimate paradoxes: Good psychological health is associated with a deluded optimism and a denial of death.

My yes-gods and my wishful thinking empowered me to take action, but I realized I needed a dose of reality as a counterpoint to my delusional thinking. I had taken on a "never say die" attitude that informed many deluded oncologists when I was in my medical training in the 1970s.

Yes, the yin needs the yang. The proverbial canary-in-the-coal mine is just as essential as the sunshine in the anteroom. That dead canary, deprived of oxygen in the deepest removes of the coal mine, provides a warning, a sentinel we ignore at our own peril. If we feel excessively hopeful and empowered, we can end up rushing headlong into our own destruction. An acute awareness of the perils we face, an acute awareness of the destructiveness of certain treatments is essential. Without this wariness we run the risk of trusting our caregivers too heavily and hastily—without taking into account the caregivers' vested interests that may or may not jibe with our own.

Ah, the wisdom of crowds, the notion that, as James Surowiecki has pointed out, a group of independent and diverse experts comes up with the wisest decision more often than any one individual. A crowd of experts balances out the biases of each separate individual. When we try to estimate the number of jelly beans or marbles in a large bowl, the mean estimate from a large group is almost always better than the estimate of any one person. Some of us may have a bias that leads us to estimate too small a number, others too large a number. A balance is essential.

Indeed boxers box, surgeons cut, radiation-oncologists irradiate—and people like me facing castration and death tend to overestimate our ability to survive and beat the odds. We are surrounded by family and friends who can become boorish cheerleaders, threatened as much as we are by the prospect of castration and death. I could not afford to deny my own death and destruction, and I would need someone to help me face the prospects of *not* beating the odds.

Contrapuntal views are essential, as I learned in my psychiatric training and in my first few years of practice. After my residency I made arrangements to obtain supervision on my most difficult cases from a controversial, older colleague. He was a brilliant man, a wunderkind who had graduated from high school at fifteen and Harvard at nineteen, a veritable Doogie Howser of his generation. Now in his fifties and in the twilight of his career, he was delighted to share his knowledge and insights with me, and he also invited me to assist him in leading psychotherapy groups. A wonderful opportunity for me since it allowed me to solidify my identity as a psychiatrist early in my career, and it allowed me to see in the flesh how a seasoned professional dealt with the most troubling psychiatric crises in real time—not just in supervision a few days later, ex post facto, in hindsight.

What also made this experience a special treat was the fact that this psychiatrist was more than a bit loony, but he came by it honestly. "Listen, Paul," he told me, "anyone who has a particular kind of intelligence that is at least two standard deviations above the norm has a capacity that sets him apart from virtually everyone else. In a sense I am like a frog who can see in color, whereas all the other frogs can only see in black and white. It can leave me with unusual perceptions and insights that others cannot understand, and it can leave me feeling different and alienated."

Not unlike the Wang sisters in China, he could see things that other mere mortals could not see.

Adding to this unique worldview was an alienation spawned by his childhood experiences. "My mother was incredibly crazy and erratic. I couldn't trust anything she said or did, and I couldn't wait to get away from the Midwest and head to college. My experiences with my mother, though, have given me a very healthy distrust of authority.

"Look at Three Mile Island a few years ago. We here in Washington were only a hundred miles from the reactor. I refused to believe anything that was coming out of the mouths of the 'authorities.' To my mind all they wanted to do was avoid any mass panic. I got on the first plane I could find and headed out to Minnesota to visit a long-lost cousin." He returned only when he could determine on his own that the Potomac coast was clear.

He continued, "if and when we do have a true nuclear disaster, I'll be one of the few survivors while the rest of you guys go through your normal wishful thinking. You'll assume that the pronouncements from the White House and the rest of the government are accurate."

Unfortunately because of his distrust of others, this psychiatrist was unable to forge meaningful long-term relationships. His pessimism and distrust and excessive self-reliance were an unmitigated detriment to survival, except under the most extreme circumstances. But he was a perfect sentinel. He had a perspective that needed to be heard, a perspective that provided a crucial counterpoint to our optimism bias, to our Pollyanna-ish worldview.

This brilliant yet daft psychiatrist taught me that a steadying hand can come from even the loopiest of sources. Just to have another perspective, a perspective that is reasonably objective and detached—though not too detached—is essential in providing a stabilizing presence in our lives. This perspective—a realistic pessimism to our excessive optimism, or vice versa—can curb our unknowing excesses. This kind of sentinel can question our headlong jumps into oxygen-depleted coal mines, and our solipsistic ruminations that have grown more fervent and bizarre with each passing day of isolation caused by illness. So what if the therapist is a flawed human being like ourselves? So what if the therapist has his own struggles and problems? Who among us does not have something overwhelming to deal with? Each of us is loopy and flawed in our own peculiar idiosyncratic ways. Should these flaws disqualify us from being able to help others overcome their flaws and wounds and diseases? There's a crack, a crack in everything; that's how the light gets in.

The healing powers may flow, not through those who have known only health, but through those who have been ill and been drawn to near death—and have then recovered. The wounded healer, from Aesculapius to Jesus.

The myth and the archetype: Aescalapius, according to Greek mythology, was plucked from death as a premature infant by his father Apollo after Apollo had killed the infant's mother for infidelity. As an adult Aescalapius became a master of the mysteries of illness and healing, of death and life. And his three daughters, Iaso, Panacea, and Hygeia became significant figures in the myths of healing as well. Their names live on in English words like "iatrogenic," "panacea," and "hygiene."

The life and after-death of Jesus followed the same trajectory as the archetypal wounded healer—death followed by a descent into the underworld, followed by a restoration to a heavenly position of healing the sick and distraught.

Not everyone who has recovered from a life-threatening illness becomes a wounded healer. Only some people, according to the myths and archetypes, are "chosen" by the gods to be healers. They are "destined" for illness so that through their illness and recovery they might be able to function as healers to a desperate and troubled mankind. That notion of a chosen people, again.

In more primitive cultures the shamanistic traditions reflect the invariable exposure that the shaman has had to the night-side of life. These experiences with a deadly or debilitating illness followed by recovery allow a person to bear witness to the mysteries and essences of life.

Men and women who have not gone through any significant reconciliation and transformation after a brush with a deadly illness— and those who have been fortunate enough to have no exposure to major illness or injury—can still be decent healers and doctors.

They can follow the protocols and the appropriate algorithms, and provide not an insignificant benefit to their patients.

Some healers, though, can be special. Take the case of Bill W. and Dr. Bob, the cofounders of Alcoholics Anonymous (A.A.) in the 1930s. The ultimate wounded healers, these guys barely snatched themselves from death and then transformed themselves through their restoration to health.

As Dr. Bob said of Bill W., "He gave me information about the subject of alcoholism which was undoubtedly helpful. Of far more importance was the fact that he was the first living human with whom I had ever talked, who knew what he was talking about in regard to alcoholism from actual experience. In other words, he talked my language." Ah, the simple wisdom of A.A. How did these two guys, a broken-down broker and a potted proctologist pull these ideas out of their butts? Just as youth is wasted on the young, A.A. may be wasted on alcoholics.

How did these guys recognize the ultimate paradox of life—that we only gain some semblance of control in our lives when we admit we have absolutely no control? A modest variation of Step One tells us, "We have admitted we are powerless over our pasts and our past traumas, that our lives have become unmanageable." To emphasize this remarkable paradox, Bill W. goes on to say, "We shall find no enduring strength until we first admit complete defeat."

Take some of the traditions from the *Twelve Traditions and Twelve Steps* of Alcoholics Anonymous:

Tradition Two: Our leaders are but trusted servants; they do not govern.

Tradition Six: An A.A. group ought never endorse, finance, or lend the A.A. name to any related facility or outside enterprise, lest problems of money, property, and prestige divert us from our primary purpose.

Tradition Seven: Every A.A. group ought to be fully self-supporting, declining outside contributions.

In these few sentences these two guys and their collaborators wiped out money and greed and pride and power and pathological narcissism—often the driving forces behind the destructiveness of human groups. Our one and only goal, they noted, is for members of A.A. to achieve sobriety—without any diverting and distracting forces.

When one adds in the efforts at making a "searching and fearless moral inventory," efforts at making "amends" to all those "we have harmed," and efforts at an altruistic "carrying" of "this message" to other fellow alcoholics, one realizes that he is in the midst of a healing brilliance. Not a literary brilliance by any means—check out Philip Roth's *Sabbath's Theater* to see a critique of the miserable literary quality—but an unusual intelligence that is as rare as that of the Wang sisters.

Their language and the program work. George Vaillant has shown that A.A. works 100 percent of the time, but slightly less than 20 percent of alcoholics avail themselves of the program in a committed way. No one with a drinking problem wants to stop drinking; with the help of alcohol, they feel no pain. All the pain is felt by spouses and partners and friends and family.

Bill W. and Dr. Bob—two schlumps who were pedestrian drunks, guys that most of us would step right over if we happened upon them at the local bus station. Hardly legendary, hardly the stuff of "Bill W. and Dr. Bob Superstars." Yet their transformation is worthy of the best transformations in all of literature. And their wounded healing is more real, less illusory and mythic, than the healing of Aescalapius and Jesus. A true life resurrection for Bill W. and Dr. Bob—and a true life resurrection for anyone who commits to the program.

The two greatest healers of the twentieth century. Contrast them with some of the twentieth-century Nobel prizewinners in Medicine or Physiology. The guy who invented the prefrontal lobotomy? How about the inventor of an alleged treatment for syphilis, by infecting the syphilitic patient with malaria? Wounded wounding, not wounded healing.

So, if we cannot trust our judgments about whom we choose as gods, if we cannot trust our judgments about who are the genuine healers in the medical sciences, how the hell can we trust our judgment in choosing a therapist?

All we can do is base it on the "fit"—our comfort level with that therapist and the confidence level we have in that therapist. Or, as Dr. Bob said, does the therapist "talk my language"?

All we can do is acknowledge our own significant flaws in judgment and the significant flaws in any and all therapists. Just as in the way we choose a god, we are all too likely to choose a punitive therapist if we have grown up with punitive parenting, or too detached and analytic a therapist if we have grown up with detached parenting.

—⁂—

Here in my hospital bed, four days after surgery in October 1984, I was realizing I needed someone, anyone—beyond my friends and family—to provide palpable therapeutic support and encouragement for my near-impossible medical mess. A psychiatric friend back in Washington, DC recognized my predicament and called the head of consultation-liaison psychiatry at the hospital I was in to come see me.

A kindly older man, the consultation-liaison psychiatrist got right to the point, knowing that he was speaking to a fellow psychiatrist. "Are you clinically depressed?" he asked bluntly after some initial pleasantries.

"Depression is not the right word for it," I muttered. "Try despair. In the past eigtheen hours since my conversation with the radiation-oncologist, even the best Chinese food brought in by my family and friends disgusts me. I cannot eat anything; I can barely sleep. All I can think about is the very recent mutilation of my pelvis and genital region with surgery. And all I can look forward to is the upcoming burning of my prostate bed through radiation—followed then by a likely death within five years, delayed only briefly and temporarily by castration. It's not a sunny scenario.

"How the hell will I *ever* be able to keep a morsel of food down ever again?" I added, with a few other expletives appended for good measure.

The psychiatrist was amiable and supportive; he provided a reasonable counterpoint to my despair and urged me to get some treatment upon my return to Washington, DC. I had already beaten him to the punch. I had called my colleague who was well-versed in the Simonton approach, to empower me in dealing with this cancer. And I called around to other colleagues to help me figure out who might be a good fit, as a plain old therapist or psychiatrist, in providing a steadying hand in my facing this cancer.

Over the years the psychiatrist whom I consulted with in Washington, DC has continued to be a genuine stabilizing and motivating presence in my life. Sure, he is a flawed mere mortal, but that mere mortalness beats a flawless, otherworldly, and illusory god any time. He has been a good fit; and, unlike the gods, he has been seeable and knowable. And he counterbalances my flawed projections and illusions, my faulty hopes and yearnings even though he, no doubt, has had his own counterprojections and illusions.

So, why did Anthony Sattilaro, in his otherwise inspiring book about his prostate cancer, not make any reference to his psychotherapy, his "analysis"—a therapy which, he acknowledged to me over the phone, had been crucial to his emotional survival after castration? Shame and stigma can be hopelessly powerful forces.

The wisdom of A.A.: "We are not responsible for our illness, but we are responsible for getting help for that illness." No self-blame, no shame, no guilt. No rational reason for us to feel we are being weak and self-indulgent in getting help. We are not being whiners and complainers; we are not wimping out. If our body has been ravaged, our mind will be ravaged. If our mind has been ravaged, it will have an effect on the viability of our body.

No need for the Cartesian mind-body dichotomy. The roots of the tree—its brains—are fully and intimately connected to the trunk and the branches and the crown and the canopy. No need for excessive and faulty self-reliance that reinforces our tendency to stay away from "shrinks." *Genuine* self-reliance—not the kind fostered by stereotypes of Horatio Alger and the Wild West—recognizes the human need to turn to others whenever life's forces overwhelm us. We cannot always pick ourselves up by the bootstraps.

Here transference again plays a role. If we have grown up with parents or others who could not help us, how can we ever assume that some veritable stranger can actually help us? Ironically, the people who are the least jaded end up receiving many of the benefits of psychotherapy, whereas the most untrusting and the most troubled human beings steer clear of the psychiatrist's consulting room.

We are all hurtling through space on a planet on which we have never lived before. It is all new to us. We cannot do it alone.

Yes, it takes a village to deal with and manage prostate cancer, and psychotherapy indeed has been a critical part of my earthly village.

If, in the wisdom of A.A., we are only as sick as our secrets, let me sing from the highest mountaintop, from the highest steeple: I would not be alive today; I would not have my testicles today if I had not gotten myself into psychotherapy.

CHAPTER 16

A Clichéd Deliverance

"We are all born for love . . . It is the principle of existence and its only end."

—Benjamin Disraeli, *Sybil*

"There is no fear in love; but perfect love casteth out fear."

—I John IV.18

"He who for love hath undergone
The worst that can befall,
Is happier thousandfold than one
Who never loved at all."

—Richard Monckton Milnes, "To Myrzha"

"Love—a grave mental disease."

—Plato

Time to sashay with a cliché. Yes, as Jorge Louis Borges has pointed out, the best metaphors are clichéd dead metaphors. Time is a river; life is a dream. And love and marriage are a union between hands and hearts.

Many writers focus on flings, brief passionate affairs, even one-night stands—unions that have not become tired and boring over time. Passion is exotic, a last tango in Paris. Grounding and stability are pedestrian and quotidian, a never-ending waltz in Topeka.

Yet how exciting is it to find a love that does not alter "when it alteration finds" as Shakespeare wrote! How exciting is it to find a partner who tackles the alterations created by prostate cancer in a marriage! How exciting is it to follow the clichés of marriage, to sustain a love through better or worse, through sickness and in health—not said just in a wedding ceremony but in the course of four decades! How exciting is it to maintain and share passions in some new and startling ways!

Is it possible to get this excitement across without exclamation points?

Enough of infatuations and flings and orgies. Enough of opera plots and so-called serious literature—none of it containing long-standing true love. Hell, in operas the love barely gets consummated. The star-crossed lover or lovers die at the end before any true relationship is realized; then the fat lady sings. Enough of the time of his or her time, the human stain going every which way, the fling that culminates in divorce and misery. Yes, all a prominent part of life—but let's see the other part: the marriage vows and marriage clichés that culminate in ongoing passion combined with a real grounding and stability.

Ups and downs to be sure, profound adjustments to be sure, passions and grounding that come and go, go and come, to be sure.

Singer-songwriters can get away with clichés. The music dilutes the clichéd wordings and allows the songs to sound more profound and idiosyncratic and exotic than they really are. But can I as a prostate cancer sufferer get away with these same clichés?

Our favorite novelists have hardly been role models for loving and long-standing relationships. Passions sell—not grounding and stability.

But clichés are valuable and real and truthful. That's why they are clichés, expressing a real human sentiment that has a universality, a relevance, a meaning for much of humanity.

So many stars have to be perfectly aligned for a long-term relationship and marriage to work—especially under intense crises. Three elements, besides luck, pulse through any ongoing relationship—desire and vulnerability and bravery. How we muster and manage all three is crucial. And when prostate cancer strikes thirteen years into a marriage, the equilibrium in those desires, in that vulnerability, in that bravery, gets smashed.

So, hats off to Helen. She has managed her desire even in the face of my months-long periods of lack of desire. What bravery— leaving herself vulnerable with me, her partner, in so many ways. In a long-standing relationship we let ourselves go, we open ourselves more fully to our partner, we put ourselves at risk for losing ourselves and losing our sense of identity. Our boundaries become more fluid as we focus on not just pleasing ourselves but also pleasing our partner. We run the risk of being swallowed up; we have put all our eggs into one basket. We become super vulnerable to losing that partner, to abandonment, especially in the face of a sex-destroying illness. No hedging our bets—so, bravery is essential. No lily-white pure Madonna partitioned off from the immodest whore—or the male equivalents, the paterfamilias partitioned off from the bad boy, the roguish gigolo, the lothario. A synthesis of the two that requires real bravery.

There may be some bravery in loving and leaving, but there is even more bravery in figuring it all out and fighting it out over time. Not just bravery, but also a capacity and willingness to manage complexity. Species that are monogamous have larger brains than those that are polygamous. Species of birds that stay with one partner have brains that can handle the complications inherent in a single relationship—the struggles, the adaptations, the demands—unlike polygamous bird species. Easier, indeed, to follow one's instincts, for males to go out and spread that seed willy-nilly; much harder to hang in there and manage the complexities.

Who knew? A big working and adaptable and flexible brain—
in both genders—may be more valuable than a big working and
adaptable and flexible set of genitalia.

Yet, with prostate cancer in the picture for Helen and me,
that knotty and naughty synthesis—that combining of a sharing
of passions along with grounding—became even more difficult, if
not impossible. How do we describe a relationship that seems to
be working, a relationship that is loving and life-giving and long-
standing, a relationship that is able to adapt, that provides this
grounding along with a genuine sharing of passions—without
invoking clichés?

I can see how someone diagnosed with metastatic prostate
cancer might say, "Okay, just castrate me, just permanently take
away my testosterone and all my androgens. Let's simplify things."
For me, though, Helen has been that crucial driving and motiving
force. Only through Helen is there this essential mantra: I will do
everything I can to retain my lust and my passions. Who cares if it
borders on lechery? Yes, so much better than sexual apathy. Yes,
let's get that stamen functioning again—working its magic on a hot
swollen pistil. Through Helen's passion I could move from being a
piece of vegetation to a man again. What powers she has had—it was
indescribable. She has brought me back to life.

Yes, I simply follow Helen's instructions, the urgings Cleopatra
gave to a messenger in Shakespeare's sexiest and most sensual play,
Antony and Cleopatra: "Ram thou thy fruitful tidings in mine ears,
That long time have been barren." The avuncular eunuch comes
back to life through Helen's urging and cajoling, Helen's loving
and not leaving. A new kind of nursemaid, a new kind of passionate
nurturing. The earth mother and the impassioned lover embodied all
in one being.

Was I putting Helen on too high a pedestal? Was I idealizing her
inappropriately—my cupid, my eros, my earth mother? Absolutely.

But I was a true believer. I believed in the sun even when it was not shining. And I believed in Helen even when the love temporarily subsided. And Helen believed in me even when I was eunichically incapacitated.

Her consistent reassurances: I will be there for you with or without our sexual relationship. I am just so happy you are here with me, you are here walking and talking and living and recovering from each and every blow. You are lucky to be alive, and I am even luckier to have you alive. An unconditional love we rarely find beyond childhood, beyond our parents' love.

Resentments were pushed to the rear. Helen and I reserved our rage and resentments for the gods, not for each other. Our terror and rage at the vagaries of the universe pulled us together. A not unheady time. A time filled with a special kind of intimacy.

To receive the explicit and implicit message that I did not *have to* regain my sexual capacities in order to be loved was lusciously liberating. It allowed me to, instead, *want to* regain my sexual capacities. No *shoulding* all over myself, as the cognitive psychologist Albert Ellis might say. I *so much wanted to* make love to Helen again and again; I did not have to.

So many shoulds in our childhood—shoulds and musts from society, from parents and teachers and coaches, shoulds from religion. All these shoulds are essential for a functioning society. But when we have adequately learned the rules of society by the age of, say, eighteen, it is time to liberate ourselves from these shoulds and have-tos. We'll follow the laws of that given society; we'll try to treat others the way we wish to be treated. But it is time to change the have-tos to want-tos, to give as much credence to our desires as to our duties.

Somehow many of us have failed to realize that we are controlled more by our inner lives and the shoulds in our inner lives than by any of the mandates from a government, from a congress, from a president. Instead, we may want to shut our own face, to change our own inner lives and all the inexhaustible shoulds in our inner lives. Even some dictatorships have fewer authoritarian shoulds and musts than our own inner lives. No more *musturbation* from someone who intermittently has been incapable of masturbation.

Helen's acceptance of my deficiencies allowed me to gain a freedom from any shoulds and have-tos, to unleash all my energies and enthusiasms and motivations to keep myself going as a sexual being, as just a being. No musts and got-tos to clog up my efforts.

In the weeks after the initial surgery, we brought our daughters on board. A marriage is not simply an extended love affair; it is also a working economic union, a means to bring the next generation into the world and begin to train them for survival and fulfillment.

We found a way to be open and honest with our then four-year-old and six-year-old daughters. No point in their hearing from their friends some weird inadvertent comments, "I heard your dad is sick," "I heard your dad has cancer," "Is your dad going to die soon?"

So, shortly after my return home after surgery, Helen and I sat down with them to discuss my medical situation—not without some intense rehearsal. Yes, guys, I do have cancer. And you do not have to live in fear of the "C" word in the way that my generation has lived. I will be able to live with cancer; our whole family will find a way to live with cancer. And cancer does not have to be a death sentence. It is a serious illness with serious implications. But I am planning to take an active stance with it, to do everything I can to deal with the disease and its treatments.

The message: Life may be different postdiagnosis and posttreatment, but that difference does not necessarily make life worse or better for us as a family, just different. I am going to face this setback in life head-on. And I hope that, whatever setbacks you may face in life, you'll be able to face them head-on as well.

Yes, "Facing it, Captain McWhirr," as Joseph Conrad puts it in *Typhoon*. "Always facing it. That's the way to get through."

For me and Helen, a remarkable moment: We had turned something potentially ruinous into a teachable moment. We had avoided the potential fiasco of secrecy. We were a lean mean fighting machine, a unit working to help me, currently its most vulnerable member, face the ramifications of prostate cancer.

Let's not forget that my daughters have been a potent and sustaining life force as much as Helen. Yet, after one has survived prostate cancer for a number of years, the heady and the heroic can become old and tired. We can fully ripen and even rot; relationships can ripen and rot. But so much better to be a ripened or even rotted old lounge singer in a Las Vegas club than to die in electrifying vibrancy at the Fillmore East.

Clichés, yes. But no irreverence or cynicism here: I love Helen so, so much; she loves me (I think). I love my daughters so, so much; they love me (I think). All is right with the world—for now (I think). I am so overjoyed to live my life as a cliché.

CHAPTER 17

A Meditation on Lust and Sex, Time and Death

Give me that man
That is not passion's slave.
— William Shakespeare, *Hamlet*

Love is a conflict between reflexes and reflections.
— Magnus Hirschfeld, *Sex in Human Relationship*

Arnost Lustig, a novelist, short story writer, and survivor of three concentration camps, was standing in front of a group of us in our living room. Helen had invited a group of colleagues and students whom she was working with at American University to come to our home to meet Arnost, to talk about literature and life. It was the early 1990s, and I was dealing with the first of many intermittent castrations.

"Fucking and eating," he boomed out bluntly. "That's how we survived the camps. That's all we thought about—what we were going to do when got out of this damn place. What we would eat and all the women we would fuck. Our imaginations were the only thing that kept us going."

Who knew? Damn, even a guy in a concentration camp had a healthier and richer fantasy life than a guy like me going through an androgen blockade. Unlike Arnost as a teenager in a concentration camp, I was no longer able to be a slave to passion. Who knew that slavery could be life-sustaining?

What a screw-job, what a double-bind, what a catch-22. We now know that the touch from a sexual relationship is more beneficial, more crucial, more life-giving for a woman with breast cancer than any other touch, than any other encounter. The touch from a sexual relationship increases oxytocin levels and a sense of attachment in a way that no other touch produces. These higher oxytocin levels and levels of attachment appear to be associated with longer survival rates.

Who knew? Damn, even women with breast cancer can experience that wonderful sexual touch in a way that a guy like me going through an androgen blockade could not.

How does a guy with prostate cancer increase his chances of greater longevity if he is denied the possibility of that life-enhancing sexual touch, a touch that is distinct from a motherly touch, from a friend's touch, from a sisterly or brotherly touch—with any sexual touch of mine or Helen's curbed by the treatment itself, curbed by the chemical castration?

How important is sex to the average adult male? Our best clue might come from our evolutionary cousin, the chimpanzee, whose more formal Latin name used to be Pan Satyrus. Here is Frans de Waal's understated scientific observation of a stable group of chimpanzees in captivity:

> It is untrue to say the life of the group is dominated by sex but this does not mean that sex is unimportant. The adult males, for example, may refuse to eat for days on end when one of the females is in her estrus period. When I see them early in the morning, in their sleeping quarters, I can read the excitement in their eyes. They have a covetous look,

which they also have when they get something especially
tasty to eat. It is clear that they are anticipating the pleasures
of the day ahead.

Perhaps Wilhelm Reich had it right all along. He was more
in touch with our inner Pan Satyrus than the rest of us. What is
the point of life without that sexual touch, without the orgasm—
or at least the promise of the orgasm? Food and sex and perhaps
some ecstatic religious experience—and very little else—have the
capacity to produce an orgasmic experience for us primates. And
even food loses its cachet in the face of sexual opportunity.

Man, I hope to get lucky tonight. And if I am incapable of acting
on my luck tonight because of an androgen blockade, I hope to get
lucky six months from now. No interest in or need for food for days
on end if I have my full complement of androgens. Ah, the hope,
the promise, the desire—all sometimes fulfilled. Ah, an intermittent
androgen deprivation—so much better than a permanent androgen
deprivation.

Only when we lose something do we appreciate its meaning
and value. Otherwise we take it for granted. Testosterone,
dihydrotestosterone, estrogen, progesterone—the sexy hormones:
We assume they will always be with us. When they are gone—damn
it, we hardly knew ye.

We men are prisoners of sex, prisoners of our hormones. Free
will?—gone as soon as we reach puberty, as soon as those hormones
start surging, as soon as we start experiencing full orgasms. As
teenagers we may think we are joining a rock band because we love
the music—partly true, but we join mostly because we want to get
laid. So too do we develop our athletic skills, our scientific chops,
our novel-writing craft, so much to respond to those sex-driving
hormones.

The timing of these testosterone surges is critical. Male rats
castrated at birth or just prior to birth fail as adults to show the mounting

behavior so typical of males in the presence of receptive females. Even if they are later given appropriate amounts of testosterone, they are incapable of engaging in this mounting behavior—the die has been cast. If these same rats are given estrogen and progesterone as adults, they assume the same sexually receptive posture as female rats in heat. Free will—gone, kaput.

Young male monkeys engage in more rough-and-tumble play than do young female monkeys—all related to testosterone levels and the effects of these levels on brain development. Among us humans young girls who have inadvertently been exposed prenatally to unusually high levels of androgens because of a congenital condition prefer the same play as boys. So, even the type of play we engage in is beyond our control.

And suppose we guys want to develop a deep baritone male voice during our teenage years and beyond. Forget about it if we happen to have a sweet and soothing soprano voice in boyhood in sixteenth- and seventeenth-century Italy. We will be castrated before puberty; we will become a castrato; we will never develop that deep male voice we may have wished for.

Timing is everything. I can vouch for the fact that any castration done after puberty will have no effect whatsoever on our regaining or retaining any high soprano voice from boyhood.

Evidence is accumulating that the timing of male hormone surges and female hormone surges may have an effect on male and female sexual orientation. Gay or straight: Our hormones—and the timing of these hormone releases—tell us who we are sexually. Free will and choice and preference have virtually no say at all.

Loss and then recovery—I was constantly playing catch-up sexually in response to prostate cancer and its various treatments. First surgery, the removal of the prostate—a nerve-sparing procedure that with time would allow the nerve tissue that feeds the genital area to recover. A loss of potency initially, a loss of jism, that creamy fluid that keeps the generations flowing, that keeps the species evolving.

And then the start of a gradual recovery. But first, radiation—6600 rads to that same fragile area. Each blow was worse than the previous one. Potency was again lost. The nerves and muscles of the pelvis were unable to move and fire. The healthy seizure-like ecstatatic quiverings of my penis dissolved in a heap. Hyperbaric oxygen gave hope that recovery was possible. Then acupuncture began to break up scar tissue—tiny needles allowed new blood vessels to form, oxygen to reach into the former prostate bed, and muscle and normal tissue to replace scar tissue. The salamander was regenerating his third leg.

Orgasmic joy, orgasmic relief. Sperm and ejaculant were gone. Fertility was gone. But potency returned. Libido was still there. My sex drive was as strong as ever. That life-giving and life-enhancing sexual touch between Helen and me kept me vibrant and aquiver. The prostate cancer was in retreat, and I was in full plumage.

The PSA test became available. My PSA was rising. Castration loomed. All the salamander's efforts at regeneration may have come to naught. My life as a man may have come to naught. Impotence, I can deal with; temporary anorgasmia, I can deal with; infertility, I can deal with; dry humping, I can deal with. But loss of lust? Castration? No way.

Intermittent castration—I can learn to live with it. The hope, the promise, the return of desire. Sign me up.

Death of the pelvis on the installment plan. Each installment was worse than the one before, but I was still standing, my penis was sometimes still standing, my pelvis was sometimes still thrusting.

But how does one regenerate after the loss of the orgasm, after castration—temporary or not? The newly blind man develops his other senses—his auditory strengths, his olfactory and gustatory senses. The newly castrated man—how does he compensate? What other senses evolve and regenerate and reverberate?

If, as W. H. Auden pointed out, lust is less a physical need than a way of forgetting time and death, then the temporarily though

repeatedly and intermittently lustless man develops a capacity
to contemplate time and death. Sex and lust may not be the most
dominant force in human and primate existence, but it is not
unimportant, says Frans de Waal. Time and death: There is nothing
more important. But we deny time, we deny death. We cannot face
them head-on.

The average adult, whether forty or sixty or eighty years old, sees
himself or herself as a twenty-five-year-old. We deny aging. Yes, we
all watch the clock. Yes, we celebrate yearly occasions—birthdays
and anniversaries and holidays. But we deny that a day has passed,
a year has passed, a decade has passed.

Instead, lust and sex distract us and allow us to forget time and
death. It can be porn, it can be fantasy, it can be *Dancing with the
Stars*—and it can be the real deal. It can be manual manipulation,
oral stimulation, genital animation. Our lustfulness heads off any
listlessness. We are alive, we can conquer the world, nothing can
stop us. Death and dying do not exist.

A seventy-five-year-old with a terminal disease—be it cancer
or heart disease or liver failure—may have no choice but to face
time and death. Yet this facing of time and death may be cut short
by death itself. But how many thirty-six-year-olds face a deadly
illness—prostate cancer—that we can possibly make into a chronic,
in some ways nondeadly, illness that gives us years to live and also
takes away lust? We have no choice but to face time and death.
Again, "Facing it, Captain McWhirr. Always facing it. That's the way
to get through," says Joseph Conrad in *Typhoon*. But most of us, with
the help of lust, do not face it. I was unable, in contrast, to forget time
and death.

A new kind of sense—a nonsexual sixth sense. A look at the
world with a different set of eyes. The masculine turns into the
feminine, the feminine turns into the masculine, the sexual turns into
the asexual, the asexual turns into the sexual—all without a sex or
gender change. No transgender, no transsexuality. The transgendered

know who they are gender-wise: We are men stuck in women's
bodies, or vice versa, they point out, but we know who we are gender-
wise. They can take the appropriate hormones to solidify that gender
identity. But how many people see their manhood or womanhood
alternate and fluctuate and mutate—and then regenerate—all in a
thirty-or-so-year period?

Yes, doesn't existence lay too much on us?

It lays too much on us, to the point that we can only contemplate
this existence, these illnesses and healings, our time and our death,
through myths and folklore and imaginary gods interacting with real
people. Aye, Aesculapius—the wounded healer—coming out of a
real womb of a real woman but fathered by a god Apollo. And his
three daughters, Iaso, Panacea, and Hygeia—all mythic figures in
the folklore of healing, all coming from a father who was snatched
from death and propelled into life.

And then there is Teiresias, the archetypal sage in Greek folklore.
Where does his wisdom come from? Walking in the forest one day, he
inadvertently or deliberately steps on two copulating snakes and hits
them with his stick. As punishment he is transformed into a woman.
For seven years he walks around as a woman until he happens upon
two mating snakes again and is turned back into a man. As a man he
becomes the wisest person in Greece, the blind seer, the soothsaying
shaman, the prophet who knows both the masculine and the feminine.

No point in looking at myths. Let's look at the reality of time
and death: when cut by a surgeon's knife, we bleed; when radiated
we burn; when faced with loss we shed real tears; when chemically
castrated we see our testicles shrink and our penises wilt.

There must be some wisdom—real, not mythic—that comes out
of that experience.

CHAPTER 18

Following the Religion of Love

"I follow the religion of Love, whichever way His camels take me."

—Sufi Muslim Sacred Saying

"We will be held to account for the joys not taken."

—*The Talmud*

It was time for me to dehypnotize myself. My hypnotic trances and my suggestibility in the face of prostate cancer allowed me to focus on my survival. A death sentence along with a hypnotic trance can concentrate the mind as no other experience can.

Sometimes we need a blow to the head, a blow to the prostate, to shake us out of cherished and strongly held beliefs—not unlike a television that needs a blow to its top to get a clearer picture, to pull it out of the fuzz and static. This blow leads to a remarkable regeneration, but not the kind of regeneration we might see in the salamander.

It is time for all of us to dehypnotize ourselves, to remove ourselves from the trances and suggestibilities of childhood. Without our realizing it, we can spend much of our adult life figuring out how to dehypnotize ourselves, to shed some of the wrong-headed beliefs that have been engrained in us in childhood, to begin to question the beliefs of our elders when those beliefs do not conform to reality, to scientific investigation, to natural experiments occurring around us. We have no choice but to believe the propaganda we grow up with—to take in and absorb and hold onto the beliefs instilled in us as children. These ideas get locked in. Rituals and traditions and celebrations reinforce these ideas, and we pass them on to future generations without questioning their validity.

Why is anyone telling us whom we can love, whom we are sympatico with, what gender we can connect with, what sexual orientation we have to follow? What authority gives anyone the right to stop any person on the planet from following the religion of Love, from going in whatever direction Love's camels take us.

Only when we look outside of ourselves and see other cultures, other views of love and sexuality, can we see the craziness of these other worldviews and by extension the craziness of our own worldview. Only when we have inquisitive anthropologists traveling to remote isolated communities—studying these communities just in the nick of time before the communities' belief systems get warped by contact with the modern world—can we see the enormous variety of worldviews adaptive for each community's special circumstances.

—m—

Love can make or break us. The meat and potatoes of any psychiatric or mental health practice is a failed love. Anton Chekhov, a practicing physician, would not be known today except for his plays and short stories about romantic disillusionment. At the same time, love can be our salvation, can save us from ourselves, can save us from our own distortions, can help us cope with the terrors of the world—the cancers, the viruses, the violence, the fluky horrors.

We now know that people can handle the stress and pain of an electric shock more effectively when someone is holding their hand.

The handling of this electric shock increases when the hand belongs to his or her partner. Neural activity in the amygdala and other areas of the brain associated with stress diminishes markedly.

When administered blisters, people recovered twenty-four hours earlier when talking with their loving partners about topics chosen to elicit supportive responses. When asked to discuss topics that provoked tension and conflict, the blisters took an extra day to heal.

Denying someone the opportunity to love, to fall in love, to sustain a love, to have a partner of either gender is like denying a man or woman food and water.

Thank the gods for the anthropologist Gilbert Herdt who, with a psychiatrist Robert Stoller—a professor at UCLA who died in a car accident in 1991—studied the Sambia people in a remote part of Papua New Guinea in the early 1970s, just before they were exposed to a more modern Indonesian world at the end of the decade. Their work, published in the *Archives of General Psychiatry* in April of 1985, just after my initial experience with prostate cancer, caught my eye. At the time, psychiatry looked at the actual whole person, not just his or her neurophysiology, but also the personal and family and cultural background—not just medication-pushing that has evolved in an era of managed care, an era in which psychiatrists have priced themselves out of the talk-therapy market.

Paradoxes abound. What makes us masculine or feminine, or super-heterosexual in the case of Sambia men and women, may have nothing to do with what Westerners conventionally consider heterosexual or homosexual, masculine or feminine. What matters is what we ascribe to our rituals or traditions, what these rituals and traditions mean to us, what message we imbue these rituals with. In a small isolated world, the entire culture buys into these beliefs and meanings, and what they ascribe and attribute to these rituals.

Once upon a time, after the heavens and earth were made, there lived a tribe of some twenty-three hundred people called the Sambia. From 1974 through 1976, when they were first studied, and then any time before 1979 when their culture began to change rapidly with the effects of modernization, they lived in a region of constant war, treacherous terrain, horrid weather, severe protein deficiency—a few possum and birds, an occasional eel to eat as sources of animal protein—periodic famine and starvation, and no medical care beyond shamans. One can hardly imagine a harsher environment for humans.

With their acceptance of the need to kill members of other tribes or be killed themselves, with their harsh circumstances creating a short lifespan, they realized perhaps thousands of years ago that they needed a great deal of luck and a great deal of feral masculinity in the men and a fierce and steady heterosexual impulse in their men and women in order to procreate and survive.

As in most cultures, close and nurturing bonds developed between mothers and their young sons in the Sambian world. Husbands and wives were forbidden to have intercourse in the first two years of their infants' lives. These wives became devoted mothers, and they focused much of their energies on their offspring while their husbands were far afield as warriors and hunters. When the sons reached the age of seven to ten, everything changed. The fathers took over the rearing of their sons. The sons were taken from their mothers and sisters; they were spirited out into the forest where their crucial secret rites of creating manhood began. At this same time, female members of the tribe were severely taboo to the male initiates, not only as erotic objects but in any other form as well.

What are these rites of passage? What is the inner life of these young boys imbued with? Let Stoller and Herdt tell this part of the story, given that the rites and the meaning of these rites are inconceivable to us Westerners.

At the height of the first-stage initiation, he (the young boy) is told the secret of Sambia maleness: One remains only the shell of a male unless he drinks as much semen as possible. He then must suck postpubertal boys' penises often, ingesting as much semen as possible during these years, for semen alone produces maleness and manliness. Because the Sambia do not believe males naturally produce semen (femaleness is the natural state), its only source (except— more or less—the milky sap or nuts of certain trees) is by taking it from other males who, in their turn, had taken it from earlier cohorts of bachelors.

The second phase began with a later initiation at around the time of puberty. The boy now has become the person sucked. From this point on, a bachelor must not fellate or suck other males. Forbidden, verboten. As Stoller and Herdt pointed out, "It (fellating other males) is taboo, for one would then be stealing semen needed by the younger boys, but, in addition, neither youths nor men report impulses to suck penises." The erotic pleasure was in being sucked; and, according to Sambian tradition, the adolescent male "nervously recognizes" that his precious semen is being depleted, that in losing semen he is losing his masculinity. He is being made less manly through this sexual release, and he believes he is gradually inching toward the femaleness from which he originally emerged.

Again, femaleness was the default position for Sambia men and women. And in his postpuberty years in adolescence, the teenage boy believed that his femaleness had come to the forefront.

For years, until he married in his late teens or early twenties, the young man was constantly having his penis sucked by the younger boys who were seven to ten years old. Until the approach of marriage and all its attendant rituals, females were taboo for these adolescents and young adults. No glances at women, no touching of the objects women use, no contact with their bodies and their secretions and their touch.

An orthodox Muslim or an orthodox Jew might not be able to create as rigid a separation of the sexes as the Sambia were able to create.

But, once the taboo of contact with women was lifted with marriage, heterosexual lust was suddenly unleashed. Heterosexuality, in fact, was the only accepted and acceptable behavior. These young men, when married, entered into intimacy with their young wives by starting with fellatio—no surprise there. Eventually the couple moved toward vaginal intercourse and full genital sexuality. Although "memories of erotically exciting fellatio" persisted for these young men, homosexuality was not an acceptable route to channel one's sexuality. Fetishism, transvestism, sadism, masochism, and anal intercourse were unknown phenomena among the Sambia—and there were no words or categories to describe these sexual activities in the Sambian language.

Despite the sexual rituals of boyhood and adolescence, homosexuality was highly negatively sanctioned. A man who persistently indulged in erotic activity with young boys would risk being called "rubbish man."

Again, Stoller and Herdt:

... the youths, when marriage approaches, start to create, without deprogramming, powerfully erotic heterosexual daydreams. And they will desire women the rest of their lives, without ever forgetting the homoerotic joys. In fact, by becoming initiators and teaching about . . . fellatio to sons and other new initiates in later years, these men are reminded and have reinforced for them the positive value of semen and homoerotic activities . . . (Nevertheless) they love their lust for women.

Only one aberrant case of genuine homosexuality among the Sambia was discovered by the two American researchers. This one man, whom Stoller and Herdt called "K."—Kafka could not have made up these sexual rites and rare deviances—had four failed marriages and almost never had any form of erotic experience with women, wives, or others. Unlike any of the other Sambia men, he was uninterested in being a warrior or hunter. His career track was that of gardening, a pursuit that his mother followed as well as many women and older men.

K.'s personal history was quite aberrant for Sambian society. His mother had had a sexual affair with a married man from a neighboring hamlet. This man ultimately rejected the mother of K. and disavowed any parental responsibility for his biological son—a highly unusual occurrence in Sambian society where male offspring were particularly desirable. Indeed there was no word in the Sambian language for a fatherless child or "bastard." This man could have taken K.'s mother as a second wife, but he refused to do so. Instead, K.'s mother became an "immoral" outcast in the Sambian world. She was condemned and beaten by her brothers as well as by others in the community. She retreated with her son to a pig herding farm "well-removed from the hamlet," in stark isolation.

K. had no male adult figures with whom to identify. With his morally offensive birth in this Sambian culture, humiliation and banishment and bastardization dominated his childhood. He grew up without a father and did not even have the benefit of his mother's brothers. He identified only with his mother and another woman with whom they lived. He was unable to establish any kind of extended partnership or intimacy with anyone, male or female.

As Stoller and Herdt wrote:

Above all else, the one act that makes no sense to the Sambia is that he (K.)—an adult—sucks boys' penises. There is no category for that. It is outside their culture and comprehension. To us (Westerners) it is a primal urge of his, a homosexual commitment based on the disasters of his childhood. He would be a homosexual anywhere, independent of the culture's erotic customs.

Me and the Sambia. The Sambian boys started out in the default feminine mode, according to the beliefs of their culture. Then by sucking teenagers' penises from age seven to ten and by swallowing as much semen as possible, they moved into a more masculine mode, only then to return to the feminine by having their penises sucked during adolescence and young adulthood—sucked by young boys no less. Then they moved into the masculine mode again when they got married and were able to indulge in heterosexual love and affection. And they were not just run-of-the-mill heterosexuals: they were super-heterosexuals—master hunters and master warriors and master lovers and master procreators.

Me and the Sambia: No, I had gained no mastery; I was anything but a master hunter and warrior and lover and procreator. But, not unlike the Sambia, I have moved back and forth between the masculine and the feminine, in similar directions but in different time frames. Ten times going from the masculine to the feminine and then back to the masculine in my adolescent and adult years.

Yet, unlike the Sambia, I did not have a cultural explanation and rationale for my going back and forth between the masculine and the feminine. My rationale was singular, that of managing a disease ready to kill me. Perhaps sucking teenagers' penises and swallowing as much semen as possible during my boyhood years could have allowed me to become a real man, a man resistant to prostate cancer, a man resistant to any need to go through temporary castrations, a man ready to handle the harsh environment of prostate cancer.

Are the paradoxes of life even thinkable? Who would have thunk that homoerotic customs in young boys would allow them, especially when indoctrinated with a specific meaning to these customs, to become "super-manly" in their adult years?

What kind of indoctrination have we been fed here in the West? "Just say no"—to sex, not just to drugs.

At least the Sambia had a set of rituals and customs for sexual initiation, even if this set of customs was outrageous by Western standards. Sexual initiation here in the West is haphazard at best. We teach our kids how to eat, how to sleep, how to read, how to pray, how to play basketball, how to maintain a household. Sex? Verboten, forbidden, especially during the childhood years. Conversations may begin in our early teenage years after we reach puberty, at best. But no rites, no rituals, no customs established when we are seven years old, when we are most hypnotizable.

Imagine our teaching our young boys diligently about sex instead of, say, religion—diligently speaking of sex when they sittest in the house, when they walkest by the way, when they liest down, and when they risest up. Imagine our male elders taking young boys and teenagers out into the local forest and teaching them how to be men, how to treat and respect women, how to treat and respect gay and straight people equally. Imagine teaching our boys and teenagers that in some cultures homoerotic rituals may lead to super-manliness and super-heterosexuality and super-procreation and—who knows?—in some cultures heteroerotic rituals could lead to nonmanliness and nonheterosexuality and nonprocreation.

At least we would be addressing sex and sexuality—and addressing it head-on as the Sambia do. None of this birds and the bees stuff, these euphemisms. We would be integrating our sexual selves into our larger lives—integrating them with playing and eating and writing and drawing and reading and singing and praying and driving and walking. Sex would not be a hushed thing, to be dealt with only at a later date, otherwise secret and mysterious—to be joked about because we really cannot talk about it in any sensible and noncontroversial way.

Here is the wily wisdom of the Sambia: They figured out a way to ritualize ejaculation and orgasm in adolescence. It would have been counterproductive to have adult men suck the teenagers' penises. That kind of ritual would have simply sanctioned and sanctified homosexuality, an accomplishment that would have thwarted the community's need for profuse procreation.

It would have been counterproductive to have teenage girls suck the boys' penises. Both the boys and girls were just getting acclimated to some major changes in their bodies, adjusting to metamorphosing from a quiescent pupal caterpillar stage, from a chrysalis to a vibrant butterfly stage. Acclimation takes time—no need to add additional excitation and confusion. And the exotic leads to the erotic: The separation of the boys from the mothers and daughters made the boys yearn for the opposite sex. Too much familiarity may lead to contempt.

It would have been counterproductive to have adult women suck the boys' penises. The adult women already had adult male partners, and procreation was moving along nicely without any glitches. Again, too much familiarity, too little exoticism.

Having children—young boys age seven to ten—be the receivers of the ejaculant is brilliant, at least in the context of a horribly harsh environment and with a belief system to match the act. You can teach these kids anything; they will believe anything; you can imbue them with a bullish belief that swallowing as much semen as possible will make them into real men. The Sambia intuitively knew of the maximal and optimal level of suggestibility and hypnotizability in young boys ages seven to ten.

And look at us here in the West. We do indeed use these years of heightened suggestibility to teach our children everything we can about our culture, customs, and rituals. Reading, writing, 'rithmetic, religious training, the four Rs—but nothing about sex. And no way to harness and use the power of the orgasm, the power of the ejaculation in our teenagers. We adults shy away from it. We joke about it. Yes, *Portnoy's Complaint, American Pie, American Reunion*—all looking at the secrecy of it, the secretiveness of the secretions. We as teenagers do not ejaculate into the mouths of seven-year-olds, but instead into cow's liver and apple pie and wads of tissues. Or into the vaginas of fellow fourteen-year-olds, not quite ready for sex, not quite ready for primetime, not nearly ready to have a baby.

And do we imbue ejaculation with any meaning, any significance—other than a possible pregnancy? Virtually none at all. Circle jerks, jerking off into the toilet, any release we guys can find. And, if we happen to grow up in a religiously fundamentalist family, we might be taught some meaning to masturbation, specifically that it is evil and taboo, that it is semen being wasted, that it is an unborn child who will never come alive, that it is potential humanity that will never come to fruition. No release is feasible at all without a huge release of guilt and shame. Masturbation as the equivalent of fetal abortion, masturbation as wasted semen, masturbation as a nascent being come to naught.

What the hell are we teaching our children? Too often nothing, too often nothing that makes sense. Too many prohibitions without enough rituals and teachings. All or nothing, sexual liberation and promiscuous pleasure or injunctions and no-no's. Mostly: let's just ignore the sex subject with our children and adolescents altogether. Certainly: no sexual initiation rites, no reasonable way of thinking about human sexuality for the twenty-first century.

And what did we Westerners end up teaching the Sambia? A new social operating system entered the picture in the last quarter of the twentieth century in the form of Christian missionaries. An extensive network of Seventh-Day Adventist and Lutheran evangelists established themselves in villages throughout the valley; and these evangelists were, in the words of Gilbert Herdt, "a remarkable force for change in sexuality and gender—offering some new role models and sometimes a form of casual sexual relationships between men and women utterly unknown to the Sambia before."

These missionaries and evangelists preached against the male ritual initiation rites and the "heathen" ways of the Sambia. The shamans and elders were often shamed and ridiculed, and attacked as "witch doctors" and "devil helpers." The missionaries also introduced Levitican-style dietary restrictions so that almost all hunting and eating of possum came to a halt. A new masculinity, based on the accumulation of Western goods, led to a migration to coastal plantations where men could earn cash in order to develop these material displays. In the meantime young women could achieve a new and different kind of status and power through schooling.

Quite a major upheaval in the social fabric within less than one generation. Fewer men remained in the villages. The women had more power and authority, with a genuine sense of equality developing between the genders. Money rather than successfully hunted possum meat became the measure of a man's masculinity and manliness. And the concept of a love or "luv" marriage became more commonplace instead of the traditional system of contracted and arranged marriages. Women were less deferential to their husbands and much less accepting of any physical abuse.

So, the modern, more civilized world has had its benefits. Exposure to a less harsh environment—with access to new foods, health care, fewer physical threats, a less isolated and brutal ecosystem—has allowed the Sambia to change their operating system. Not to change easily and comfortably—but to change nevertheless, and in a quicker way than one can imagine people in the West changing.

Has not the operating system, the mental and religious software, the signposts on our doorposts and our gates here in the West also run its course?

With the advent of the industrial revolution, of the information age, of the knowledge-based economy, of the nuclear age, we here in the West are still stuck with a belief system that formed twenty-seven hundred years ago with the Old Testament, nineteen hundred years ago with the New Testament, and fourteen hundred years ago with the Koran. What we teach our children is outdated and bizarre, as strange in its own way as what the Sambian elders taught their children.

With my prostate cancer I wanted to believe in the Sambian way of thinking. Yes, the masculine to the feminine to the asexual to the emasculated and back to the masculine. The heathen in me told me that I must not have sucked enough penises, swallowed enough semen in my malleable and suggestible childhood years. If only I had known: I would have been delighted to have fellated hundreds of adolescent boys, even thousands and millions of teenage boys—*if* I could have believed that sucking the penises of these teenagers would have made me more of a man, *if* I could have believed it would allow me to retain or regain my seminal fluids and sexual juices.

But, alas, I could not believe any of the Sambian nonsense, nor could I believe much of the nonsense coming out of the sacred texts of Judaism and Christianity and Islam.

I could believe the following: that up was usually up, but sometimes up was down; that masculine could be feminine; that gay could be straight; that left could be right; that our universe is more mysterious and paradoxical than any of the ancients could have realized.

Do we really need a purely heterosexual world in the twenty-first century? Unlike the Sambia pre-1975, we are not living in a brutal and harsh environment in which a feral masculinity is essential. Unlike the world in biblical times, we understand the universe a bit more; we understand the value and meaning of a "luv" bond a bit more; we understand gay and straight a bit more; we understand the bonds of sex and love a bit more.

To survive I follow the religion of Love, wherever His camels take me. My seminal vesicles have been ousted; my prostate has been discarded; my androgens have periodically been ablated. But I can still follow the religion of love.

How can any of us deny love, the perks of love, the boons of love to another couple, to any other couples—based on an outdated belief system from millennia ago?

For any of you adults out there—men and women, gay or straight, transgender or not—a warning: Please make use of your genitals— yes, responsibly and consensually. We only recognize the value of things when we lose them. Teach your children to enjoy adult sexual play and the bonds of love before it is too late.

A man without a prostate, a man without seminal vesicles, a man without androgens—I can think of worse things to reconcile oneself to. But I cannot, for the life of me, think of too many worse things.

CHAPTER 19

Sermons in Stones, Clarity in Calamity, Cogency in Cojones: Rebooting and Regenerating My Inner Life–and the Collective Inner Life

"Men make use of their illnesses, at least as much as they are made use of by them."

Aldous Huxley

"Sweet are the uses of adversity,
Which, like the toad, ugly and venomous,
Wears yet a precious jewel in his head;
And this our life . . . Finds tongues in trees, books in the running brooks,
Sermons in stones . . ."

William Shakespeare, *As You Like It*

I have now faced the nightside of life, happily and unhappily, for the past thirty years. One of the benefits of prostate cancer, at least mine, is the longevity it has given me. In facing this nightside for an extended period, we prostate cancer stragglers have time to say long good-byes to our friends and family, and to look at life in all its vagaries and hypocrisies. Unlike victims of wars and holocausts and many diseases—heart disease and cancers like melanoma come to mind—I have not gone to my end, to the slaughter quickly. I have lingered; I have seen things that others may not see. A new kind of salvation, of redemption, of regeneration.

I did not ask to see these things; I did not want to see these things. Like every mortal I wanted to believe in my immortality, to deny my fragility, to negate the existence of illness and death. I wanted to keep playing tennis three times a week, to do the work I love; I wanted to raise my family, to love Helen, and to love my two daughters. To make love to Helen. *Ego diligam, ego sum; Amo, ergo sum; coito, ergo sum.* "I love and will love, therefore I am; I fornicate, therefore I am. A new variation of *cogito ergo sum.*

Prostate cancer has created a new reality; it has taken me away from my previously unacknowledged delusions and denials; it has forced me to transform my inner life. In my efforts to restore my sexual health and to extend my life, I have managed to reboot my brain and see life through a new lens.

Yes, life can be extended; sexual health can be extended. If I as an individual can achieve this extension, so can we generalize to us as a species. Every species, just like every living cell, is programmed to die. We human beings are the only species programmed, through our scientific knowledge and our ability to create lethal tools, to be capable of killing off our own selves. But there are ways of extending our life as a species and prevent us from destroying ourselves prematurely.

The key lies in our collective inner lives, which as reflected in our religions, have become stale. Our inner lives have not kept pace with the experiences and knowledge and collective wisdom that have accumulated in the past few hundred years. Given the staleness of our religions, we have no way of reconciling religion and science. No new shared or unified visions have come forth since the writing of the Koran and the New and Old Testaments.

We have taught the ideas and rules articulated in these books all too diligently to our children for at least a hundred generations. For many centuries these books were the only texts in print. Most people were illiterate. Scribes, among the only few who were literate, became highly valued for their ability to bring these texts into being.

These books served a vital purpose. For Jews the Torah, or the five books of Moses, reached a higher level of sanctity after the development of Christianity. Before Jesus's apotheosis Jews were not viewing themselves as the "people of the book." But with the evolving popularity of Christianity throughout the Mediterranean, the Jews were tormented. They lost their identity in the face of a new religious movement. Interpretations of the Torah through Talmudic and rabbinical study and debate became a way of life for literate Jews over the course of many centuries—in a variety of settings including Judea and Samaria, Babylonia, Spain, and Eastern Europe. They retreated from the world, and the Torah became their organizing and motivating force, the major source of their identity.

The book became a fetish, an obsession, an idol. Even in the twenty-first century, on every Saturday, Jews worship the Torah as if it were a god itself—kissing it at Sabbath services, hugging it as if it held their salvation, parading around with it in paroxysms of joy and tribulation. Idol worshiping ironically at its worst, for a people who originally created their religion as a way of eliminating idol worship.

In a similar way Jesus and Christianity became an organizing and unifying principle for most of the Mediterranean and on into all of Europe. Christianity's own book, the New Testament, became a source of laws and values, but at the same time the very conception of Jesus, the notion of the virgin birth, served to negate and corrupt human sexuality. The notion of Jesus as a Son of God gave life to an anthropomorphic god, with a view of a palpable god made in the image of man and a view of man made in the image of god. More idols emerged in the form of Jesus and Mary.

Six centuries after the arrival of Jesus and after the Jews retreated from the political world into their books and laws, the Arabian world was transformed by the Koran. The Koran was the first major book written in formal Arabic, and this formal language took hold as a unified way of expressing the Arabic language in written form. Without the Koran the spoken Arabic languages would have remained splintered with diverse dialects from region to region—a phenomenon still in existence to some degree today.

The Koran indeed has served a significant purpose in bringing together a diverse world from northern Africa to the Middle East and to the Saudi peninsula. The book has provided a unifying principle for propagating the impressive spread of Islam throughout Asia and Africa, into Indonesia and southern Africa in the past century.

Any book that has the power to shape a language also has the power to shape the inner life, the thought processes, the values of an entire culture.

With the arrival of Gutenberg and the printing press over five hundred years ago, we might have expected the possibility of making books other than bibles. But the initial impetus was to spread The Word, to produce more and more bibles. Ironically, with the advent of printing, the imprint on our brains and on our inner lives from these so-called sacred books became even greater. Translations of these texts into numerous languages made the new editions accessible and palpable. Everyone on the planet potentially became a person of The Book—whatever book we were exposed to as children. If we were illiterate, unable to read the book, we could at least memorize passages in this designated book. The ultimate imprint, the ultimate propaganda machine.

And the propaganda has always had purpose: to preserve the life of the larger community, the group in which one belongs—even if it means that the individual in that group sacrifices himself in his willingness to die for his community and to die for his god.

Contrary to popular belief, religions do not cause wars or crusades. No, wars cause religion; wars are the midwife of religion. Wars and our warring nature create a need for religion, a need for a god to inspire us to kill and be willing to be killed. Human bellicosity— it's all in our nature—requires religious fervor, something to inspire us to go to our death in the face of battles with our enemies, with the outsiders, with the alien group—something to make us willing to kill others despite our capacity for compassion and empathy, something to make us willing to destroy another group or society or community despite the prohibitions against killing in our civil and religious laws.

Yes, my god is better than your god. My book is better than your book. My scriptures—my blueprint and owner's manual—are better than your scriptures. My love of my god is fuller and richer than the love you have for your god. I am part of the chosen people; you are not one of the chosen. I am faithful to my god; you are an infidel. I will go to heaven; you will rot in hell. My god will bless me in life and in death; my god will curse you in life and in hell for your godlessness.

Chances are Moses never existed, as Nicholas Wade has noted in *The Faith Instinct*. He was created as a figure to help inspire an effort to unite two small kingdoms, Israel and Judah, in the seventh century BC, after the Assyrians had withdrawn from the region. The notion that the Israelites had lived in Egypt and escaped from Egypt three hundred years earlier may have been pure fiction.

Jesus was a small figure prophesizing a catastrophe unless his fellow Jews changed their ways—a small figure made larger than life by the Christ movement three hundred years after his death.

Mohammed probably never existed other than as a word drawn out of a gerundive phrase referring originally to Jesus— *"muhammadun rasul allah,"* meaning "The messenger of god is to be praised." "Muhammadun" is a gerund, meaning "one who should be praised." Centuries later this phrase, now a key statement of the Muslim faith, is translated as, "Muhammad is the messenger of God." In the seventh century, Arabian-Christian rulers were attempting to separate themselves from the Christ movement and from the notion of a holy trinity; instead, Jesus alone was to be praised. The Koran may have been derived from the Syriac Christian liturgical work—note the inscriptions on the Dome of the Rock in Jerusalem, including "For the Messiah Jesus, son of Mary, is the messenger of God." Ultimately, around the year 575, the Arabian-Christian tribal leaders of the Near East and North Africa were overthrown by the Abbasids who separated themselves further from Syriac Christianity. They made Mecca the holy city instead of Jerusalem or Damascus, and the Koran was reinterpreted and reimagined as a new text for a new religion. This text and religion provided a unifying identity for these new Arab rulers and for their subjects to help in the fight against the Byzantine empire next door.

Monotheism is a joke. Based on folklore, myths, fiction, and occasional true events—who can tell what is true, what is made up?—the books are a joke. Yes, they have some inspiring stories; they will always be part of our canon. But do they have to continue to light the fuse for our nuclear cannons? The natural order of things has changed dramatically in the past seventy years with the development and evolution of nuclear power and nuclear weapons. If the anthropomorphic gods—a separate god for each religion— inspire us to light the fuse of a nuclear bomb, our species as we know it comes to an end.

To paraphrase the old Soviet Nikita Khrushchev, "The survivors (of a nuclear war) would envy the dead."

Monotheism served its purpose. A breakthrough in human thinking at the time of its inception twenty-five hundred years ago, a breakthrough in the human capacity to think abstractly instead of concretely, monotheism has outlived its usefulness. It helped unify disparate peoples; it provided inspiration to allow people to fight and die for the survival of their people. The initial monotheism, Judaism, helped a group of people survive when surrounded by hostile forces, the Egyptians and Assyrians, on either side, to survive subsequent expulsions and diasporas and holocausts. A second monotheism, Christianity, helped to unify people throughout the Mediterranean, then into northern Europe, parts of Africa and Asia, eventually into the New World. A third monotheism, Islam, helped to unify the Middle East, much of Africa and Asia, all the way to Indonesia.

But enough, already. Enough of a punitive god created twenty-seven hundred years ago—a god that, according to the first of the ten commandments, is an unusually and pathologically narcissistic god who does not want his name taken in vain, an anthropomorphic god who responds as angrily as a kid on an urban street corner when the kid's name is taken in vain. Enough of a god that creates his son asexually, through an immaculate conception, a god and a son whose very conception has corrupted human sexuality. Enough of a god whose prophet is actually a gerund, whose people are praising and worshiping a gerund and going to war on behalf of this gerund. A gerund.

Indeed, as Voltaire pointed out, "God is a comedian, but he's playing to an audience too afraid to laugh."

In a nuclear age our inner lives have no choice but to go through a transformation, to recognize the potential self-destructiveness of a god who inspires us to got to war, who inspires us to use all of the weapons at our disposal, even if those weapons destroy us in the process. Our warlike nature creates the need for religion: Religion does not cause wars, but it does provide a reinforcement for war in a forceful feedback loop. It unifies people, and then separates them from other people and reinforces our natural xenophobia, our fear of the outsider who then is seen as less than human, as godless, as a pagan.

And who could have predicted that the QWERTY phenomenon would have affected and locked in ideas, not just affected and locked in typewriter keyboards and tufted carpets? The QWERTY principle, as outlined by the economic historians Paul David and Brian Arthur in the 1980s, describes how easy it is, say, for a typewriter keyboard design to get locked in for over a hundred years by the accidents of history. Originally designed so that typists would type slowly on machines that could easily jam, the QWERTY keyboard has not been easy to displace with better designs mainly because these new designs have not been stunningly better than the QWERTY design. For well over a century, typists have learned to type on a QWERTY keyboard, and manufacturers continue to make QWERTY keyboards because typists demand them. We have a feedback loop that has allowed the QWERTY keyboard to take on a life of its own, even in an age of computers and nonjamming keyboards.

To apply economic jargon, the QWERTY phenomenon produces an "external economy of scale." After World War II American carpet production became concentrated in the small town of Dalton, Georgia, because of a simple accident of history. A teenage girl in Dalton in the late nineteenth century had produced a tufted bedspread that became the prototype for tufted carpeting eventually displacing woven rugs in the mid-twentieth century. The handicraft skills that she and her colleagues developed became essential for the production of tufted carpets. As tufted carpeting took hold, a virtuous circle for Dalton took hold. People with the necessary handicraft skills moved to Dalton. They were assured of work, and the companies that produced the product were assured of expert labor.

Similar feedback loops and virtuous circles have occurred in Silicon Valley and in the Route 128 corridor near Boston in the computer industry—and in Benton, Arkansas, where Sam Walton's presence spurred a cottage industry of suppliers for Wal-Mart. Likewise in Bangalore and Hyderabad in India.

Most of these QWERTY phenomena are harmless and even beneficial—except in the case of the religion industry. An accident of history, not unlike the appearance of a tufted bedspread innovator in Georgia, brought the writers of the Old Testament, the New Testament, and the Koran—along with their fictional or real characters, Abraham, Moses, Jesus, Paul, John, and Mohammed— into a close geographical proximity. Now this limited geographical area supports a wide network of purveyors of religion, a populous pool of skilled labor. Rabbis, mullahs, imams, ministers, and priests gravitate to this Middle Eastern religious mecca. Yeshivas, madrassahs, and bible schools thrive with the help of government subsidies. Places like Jerusalem and Bethlehem and the Sea of Galilee and Medina and Mecca and Karbala and Najaf draw religious ideologues from all over the world in a phenomenon that the journalist Edward Fox has called "negative cosmopolitanism," a sense that one can and should live there and only there rather than anywhere else in the world.

Enough, already. It's time to disentangle religion and spirituality from the badlands and deserts and rubble of the Middle East. This whole planet is sacred. A sense of wonder, a sense of the strangeness of our world and our universe, a sense of the supernatural can arise anywhere.

Oil and holy water do not mix. Oil and religion do not mix. Our old religions and a nuclear world do not mix. Our old religions and our current scientific understanding of the universe do not mix.

The gods are not dead. Religion and faith and spirituality are not dead. Instead, our vision of an anthropomorphic god—a god who rewards us and punishes us, who selects us as the chosen ones, who settles scores with our foes—is in its final agonizing death throes. We can begin to recognize the wisdom of Carl Jung's line, "Religion is a defense against genuine religious (that is, spiritual) experience."

Our world is a stranger and more surreal place than the ancients had any clues about. We do not have to invent a supernatural connection between us and the universe. We do not have to invent a Moses as a prophet from God, reshape a mere mortal like Jesus into a Son of God, or believe that an angel from god dictated and created a sacred text like the Koran.

No, the angels and the gods, not just the devil, are in the details.

—◠—

I am not a physicist. Most of the us on this planet are not physicists. Yet most of us know that our base of knowledge has changed in dramatic ways over the past century. The disparity between our collective knowledge and our faiths is wider than ever before.

In 1927, as quantum theory was getting off the ground, the famed physicists Wolfgang Pauli and Werner Heisenberg shared their concerns about this disparity. "It's all bound to end in tears," noted Pauli. "At the dawn of religion, all the knowledge of a particular community fitted into a spiritual framework, based largely on religious values and ideas. The spiritual framework itself had to be within the grasp of the simplest member of the community. . . . If he himself is to live by these values (the underlying community values), the average man has to be convinced that the spiritual framework embraces *the entire wisdom of his society* (emphasis mine). . . . The complete separation of knowledge and faith can at best be an emergency measure, afford some temporary relief . . ."

Yes, the gods are in the details. The gods—the supernatural— may lie in the quanta.[1] Atoms emit energy only in discrete amounts or "lumps" called quanta (from the Latin word for "how much") rather than in the continuous waves prescribed by electromagnetic theory. The quantum is a bundle of energy, possibly an indivisible unit that we currently believe cannot be sliced any further. Light behaves as if it were composed of these little energy bundles. And, if

1. The Higgs Boson has been called the "God particle," but it might more accurately be called the "Goddamn Particle," as noted by the Nobel Prize–winning physicist Leon Lederman, commenting on its elusiveness and the amount of resources spent on trying to find it. What appears to be its presence was confirmed in July, 2012, at the CERNS Collider outside of Geneva, Switzerland.

light as a wave can be a particle or bundle, then conversely particles can also be waves.

The problem is that particles do not always end up where something called wave function—developed in an equation by Erwin Schrodinger in 1925—predicts they will end up. When electrons are measured and observed, they usually are situated in the most likely place, but they are not guaranteed to be in that place, even though this wave function can be calculated quite precisely. We can expect certain probabilities, but they are merely probabilities. Nothing is certain. So much is open to the music of chance.

As the English writer and prince of paradox, G. K. Chesterton, pointed out, "The commonest kind of trouble is that it (this world of ours) is nearly reasonable, but not quite . . . It looks just a little more mathematical and regular than it is; its exactitude is obvious, but its inexactitude is hidden . . ." Hidden in the quanta.

From quantum theory has come the complementarity principle. Niels Bohr noted in this principle that, although light is both a particle and a wave, an experimenter or an observer can measure one aspect or the other but not both at the same time. Complementarity and contradictions rule the universe. Ironies and paradoxes rule the universe. Matter leads us to antimatter.

Two decades ago two teams of physicists managed to make current go in two directions at exactly the same time around tiny superconducting loops of wire. Electrons and photons can be pictured, as the physicist Richard Feynman pictured them, as getting from point A to point B by taking all possible pathways at once. Only by observing the electrons in one discrete moment in time can we determine which pathway they took.

So, particles can be everywhere and a specific somewhere at the same time. The world can follow a course of smoothness and steadiness and at the same time a course of quantum fluctuations. Particles can be waves, and waves can be particles. The real and the unreal can coexist. The classical world can coexist with a quantum blur.

Do we need to create anything more spooky and mysterious than what the universe already is?

Even Albert Einstein never entirely got it, never was able to fully put his arms around the weirdness of the universe: "It is hard to sneak a look at God's cards. But that he would choose to play dice with the world . . . is something I cannot believe for a single moment." Hey, Alberto, get with it. The gods, the quanta, are the very dice you speak of. At some point, however, he did admit that "something deeply hidden had to be behind things."

—◆—

The Bible, the New Testament, the Koran are not going away—but do they have to continue to be such a strong part of the canon for our children? At our most suggestible and hypnotizable age, our elders expose us to stories about a big man in the sky who rewards us for good behavior, who delivers horrifically harsh punishments for bad behavior—floods and pestilence and the deaths of the firstborn—a god whom *The Onion* once headlined as having been diagnosed with bipolar disorder. His periods of manic wrath are terrifying.

We know why this god and his prophets are always male. Yes, war is the midwife of religion. So, testosterone is the fuel for war; testosterone is the fuel for a willingness to go to war and to one's death; testosterone is the fuel for male-centric religions that inspire us to go to our death for the sake of our god and our community. Bad behavior is defined as an unwillingness to serve that god. In our heightened suggestibility we become servants, indeed obsessive slaves, to that god.

As the sciences continue to expose the strangeness of our universe, religion will need to reflect that weirdness. No more of the conventional tales and rules, and males, that have previously explained our world. We have moved on to the larger cosmos, a much larger, less parochial neighborhood. As our universe expands, as we learn more about possible parallel universes, as we come

to understand the finiteness and infiniteness of our universe, the finiteness and infiniteness of possible multiple universes, our inner lives can begin to expand.

Is it possible to be a deist, albeit a skeptical and cynical deist a la Voltaire, in this present world? You bet it is. We can pray to the gods, to the quanta, to the electrons, to the photons, to the light and the darkness as easily as ever before. Prayer makes even more sense than ever before. With prayer we are removing ourselves from the daily grind; we are stopping our world at one moment in time. We are observing the quanta at that one specific moment in time; we are allowing ourselves to see the light moving along one specific pathway, not along infinite pathways. We are able to contemplate and see the specific space we are in; we are able to contemplate and see what velocity we are traveling in. And we are trying to find a way to influence and move the quanta, the electrons, the photons in a direction that gives us the greatest chance of good health and contentment and occasional moments of joy.

Yes, pray to the quanta, pray to the gods: Hear, O people of this Earth, the Lord is *not* One. They, the gods, the quanta are infinite and finite at the same time. The gods are ineffable; the gods are invisible; the gods are unimaginable; the gods are undelineable. These gods are not made in man's image. Man is not made in these gods' images. These gods are not made in a raccoon's image, nor in the image of any other animal.

There is no chance that the gods follow the patterns of human social hierarchies. There is no "our Father, our King." The gods cannot have sons. The gods do not send down prophets and angels from the heavens.

It will be terrifying to give up the *old* God, the old big guy in the sky, the old prophets, the old books and scriptures—or to at least give up the sacredness of these books and scriptures. Change is always frightening. Familiarity always trumps unfamiliarity. The god and devil we know is better than the god and devil we do not know, we tell ourselves. The old God and books have been organizing and stabilizing and motivating forces for hundreds of years. We cannot underestimate how difficult it will be to give up these ideas and beliefs.

At the same time, it is crucial to realize how far our species has come in the last few hundred years. We are no longer in a Malthusian trap. We are no longer in a zero-sum game in which people's deaths allow others to survive; we are no longer in a world in which limited food and resources require us to kill so that others of us may live.

We have civil laws that carry as much weight and authority as religious laws have carried in the past. We do not need sharia, we do not need halakhah—we do not need the belief that the laws have come down from a god in order to give these laws the authority they need. Religious laws, particularly the laws from European Catholicism almost a millennium ago, gave us a running start—and now we can begin to move on.

We have begun in the past two hundred years to create civil societies that give men and women the respect and opportunities they deserve. We have gotten rid of slavery; we are getting rid of gender biases; we are getting rid of discriminations against people representing minority differences—whether of skin color or religious upbringing or sexual orientation.

We have begun to design punishments that actually fit the crimes. We do not need divinations from a higher power to determine what is right and what is wrong, what is punishable and what is acceptable in a reasonable and just society. We have moved beyond a *Lord of the Flies* mentality to a more adult-like view of the world: Our punishments for actual crimes are less frantic, more just, and more fair than those of the ancients, than those prescribed in the ancient texts. No more need for shipwrecked twelve-year-olds to determine the rules of the game.

Our capacity to put in place first-rate leadership, at least in the West, has improved in the past two hundred years. And our capacity to remove leaders who are corrupt, leaders who are demagogues, has improved as well. We no longer need leaders whose authority flows

from a presumed connection with the gods, whose royal trappings
are linked to the gods. We have matured as a species. We know toxic
leadership and good leadership when we see it—even if we are at
times unable to change that leadership.

One of the elements that locks in our beliefs in the old God—the
big guy in the sky—is our natural suggestibility and hypnotizability
as children. As noted earlier, this suggestibility is on the rise in
early childhood until its peak at age nine, then tails off until the
age of nineteen, at which time it virtually disappears. So, when the
Abrahamic faiths command us to teach our children diligently about
this one God, about the teachings of this one God, about the rewards
and punishments emanating from this one god, we are undeniably
hooked. For us as children the notions of God, and the stories from
the old texts get drilled into us at a time when we are the most open
and most vulnerable and most hypnotizable. We get locked in. We
get indoctrinated. It all sticks. Yes, time to dehypnotize ourselves.

On top of this suggestibility lies our concrete thinking before
the age of twelve. Indeed, our capacity to think in abstract terms
only begins to develop at the age of twelve and thereafter. At a
time of heightened suggestibility, we can only think of a god in
purely concrete terms, in purely anthropomorphic terms. Without
literal concrete idols to serve as stand-ins for the gods, we create as
children, a vision of a god that is just as concrete as any idol. We get
locked in to that vision.

When facing any struggles, any sense of helplessness as adults,
we return to that vision of an anthropomorphic god—a god who can
even have a son. When coming to grips with our own fragility, we
return to that vision of a god who will save us and protect us and
take care of us—not just in this life but also in the afterlife. With
a kind of wistfulness as we age, we return again and again to a god
that seemed to make the world a more innocent place when we were
children. We yearn for our old innocence that allowed us to see the
world as a more reasonable and exact place than it really is.

A changeover in our conception and understanding of the gods is inevitable. Just as we human beings are waves and are riding certain waves, so are religions riding certain waves. Apoptosis: Every living cell is programmed to die, to be replaced by a new, more vibrant cell. Every human being is programmed to die, to be replaced by a new, more vibrant human being. The ancient religions are programmed to die, to be replaced.

When apoptosis is eliminated and denied, cancers develop; pure destruction and death ensue. Apoptosis is the fuel for creative destruction—the new replaces the old. Every organism is programmed to die. No point in extending life unnecessarily, no point in making the eighty-something into a ninety-something, and no point in making the ninety-something into a centurion. The new replaces the old; new ideas replace the old ideas. A new kind of Malthusian world in which the older cells and organisms die so that the newer ones can live.

When the old religions die, we can only hope that it is a less than violent death. We cannot expect the current religion industry to help in any way in this transformation. The pastors, the imams, the rabbis—as well as university theology departments—have a vested interest in maintaining the status quo. They study the past; they study every line of scripture; they study every conceivable interpretation of the ancient texts. Their very livelihood depends on sustaining the QWERTY keyboard of the ancient religions.

So many vested interests in keeping the status quo: our religious schools, our religious training in childhood, our suggestibility, our concrete thinking in childhood, our yearning for a lost innocence.

The Sambia, for better or worse, were able to give up their ancient beliefs, their modus operandi, in one generation. We may need several generations; we all may need to die off and die off and die off. Our ancient collective wisdom will then die off, slowly and then more quickly. A phase reaction picking up steam—all inevitable. At some point these Abrahamic faiths will look like historical artifacts—a fraternity or sorority, an ethnic or religious group that carries much less meaning than it does currently.

This change in the way we imagine our gods will be difficult. The Scopes trial—and the resistance to the concepts of Darwin and evolution—may look like child's play compared to the changeover in our conception of the gods. The legendary smashing of idols by Abraham—in the face of resistance to a belief in a more abstract god—may look like child's play compared to this coming changeover.

The danger in this transformation lurks when "fresh knowledge threatens to explode the old spiritual forms," as Wolfgang Pauli reminds us. Yet this change will be liberating. We as a species will be liberated from a punitive and narcissistic god. We will be liberated from rules and commandments that may have made sense hundreds of years ago but make little sense now. We will be free to be our true selves, free from unnecessary and unwanted shame and guilt. We can be straight, we can be gay, we can be transgender; we can be healthy, we can be sick; we can be busy living and busy dying—all without feeling that some god has visited upon us a reward or punishment for some presumed sin of omission or commission.

No panacea in any of this—but a better meshing of science and religion, of our collective knowledge with our faith. No brave new world of reasonable and sensible and caring people. The insensitive and cold-hearted bastards will still be trying to take over the world; the drunken drivers will still have the right of way. But our illusions can be more in check; our willingness to face the reality of our weird universe will be enhanced.

Quantum theory tells us that the connection between cause and effect is not as clear-cut as we had previously come to believe. How liberating to disconnect our unfounded guilt, as well as our unfounded shame and embarrassment and self-consciousness, from the events unfolding around us. We can liberate ourselves from an all-seeing and all-knowing anthropomorphic god who is looking down at us and watching our every move, who is determining whether we are acting in a good way or bad way.

Enough of a micromanaging god.

Life is difficult enough with lurking pathogens and lurking genetic deviations and lurking personal misunderstandings and lurking personal conflicts. Why add another layer of strangeness with a set of ideas that do not fit with our current understanding of psychology and biology and chemistry and physics and cosmology? Why add another layer of strangeness with a set of childlike beliefs in a single god, a monocracy, a monolithic and anthropomorphic deity, a monotheism that can only lead to our own destruction?

We do not have to spend our energies serving—at times being slaves to—each of the punitive and narcissistic gods of the Abrahamic faiths. Our governments do not have to subsidize religions and religious schools. We will have more time and resources to spend with our families and our communities; we will have more energy to allow ourselves to have fun and be productive. Economists have shown that a society that spends less time and resources in serving the gods has a more productive and fulfilling society. Medical researchers have shown that a person with a disease has a better prognosis, a better response to treatment if he does not believe his disease is a visitation from a punitive god.

With a renewed view of the gods, we can accept, instead of fight, the complementarities and the contradictions of life. We can begin to be startled and astounded by the paradoxes and ironies of life. We can begin to see good and evil in new ways. With every curse lie the seeds of a blessing. With every blessing lie the seeds of a curse. Every particle is a wave, and every human being is filled with particles that are waves. All we can do is ride those waves—and perhaps stretch or contract those sine waves. Free will and necessity, free will and predetermination, all at the same time.

Yes, the yin and the yang, the West and the East, the North and the South, matter and antimatter, expansions and contractions, smoothness or steadiness and quantum fluctuations, the predictable and the unpredictable. Particles can be everywhere and some specific somewhere, all at the same time. Good and evil, all at the same time.

Irony of ironies. Complementarities abound all around us. Hitler and Stalin brought the world closer together. Hirohito in Japan brought the Eastern world in to follow along. It was not called a world war for nothing.

And "the real father of the atomic bomb (and atomic energy) was Hitler and the specters his horrifying will conjured up," noted the historian Paul Johnson. Fear was the primary motive for harnessing atomic and nuclear power. Robert Oppenheimer, a Jew, led the frantic effort in Los Alamos, New Mexico, to build the first atomic bomb because he feared Hitler would do it first. Edward Teller, a Hungarian, was instrumental in building the first hydrogen bomb out of horror over Stalin's immense Soviet terrorism.

So, thank you, Adolph. Thank you, Joseph. The terror you generated has stretched us, forced us to face a brave new nuclear world, confronted us with quanta and photons and bosons—newly discovered invisible and indivisible gods—that we ignore at our own peril.

So, thank you, even to the perpetrators of 9/11: The three thousand people they killed on September 11, 2001, have not died in vain. The appalling actions of the perpetrators have unleashed a realization in much of the rest of the world that each of the literalist and fundamentalist Abrahamic faiths—not just Islam—has reached the end of the line. Atheists have been able to come out of the shadows. We can hear more talk of the "god delusion" and of god not being "great." We can recognize the wisdom of the comments of Yitzhak Rabin just before he was killed by a fundamentalist Jew in Israel, that the conflict is not between Jews and Muslims, between Muslims and Christians, between Christians and Jews, but between fundamentalists and secularists.

Or, perhaps it is between fundamentalists or literalists and a new kind of deist. Let's listen to the British philosopher Isaiah Berlin:

Because the ram duly grows fatter, and perhaps is used as a bell-weather for the rest of the flock, he may easily imagine that he is the leader of the flock, and that the other sheep go where they go solely in obedience to his will. He thinks this and the flock may think it too. Nevertheless the purpose of his selection is not the role he believes himself to play, but *slaughter* (italics mine)—a purpose conceived by beings whose aims neither he nor the other sheep can fathom.

We are just as lost and as clueless as that ram and the sheep that follow him. And our efforts to cling to the certainties and supposed verities of our ancient texts will make us only more clueless—in a nuclear world, no less.

So, let us experience gratitude and terror at the same time. Gratitude at the wonders of nuclear energy and the modern world it has created, and terror at its potential to destroy our entire species. With the first atomic bomb over southern New Mexico, we witnessed heat and temperatures that were four times more intense than those generated at the center of the sun. The harnessing of this atomic and nuclear energy has stopped some prostate cancers in its tracks. And nuclear energy run amok has awarded us with the countermeasure of hyperbaric oxygen.

Gratitude at the wonders of testosterone and the ingenuity of the human world that testosterone has fueled—and terror at the bellicosity and wars it has fueled. The raping and pillaging it has fueled. The prostate cancers it has fueled. Perhaps going from the masculine to the feminine and back to the masculine, a la the Sambians, can save us.

Gratitude to the sacred texts—and the gods of the Abrahamic faiths—for their ability to unify disparate peoples, for their initiation of laws and ruliness in the midst of lawlessness and unruliness. Terror at the disparity between our current scientific knowledge and the notions conveyed in these sacred texts. Terror at the monotheism that fuels the notion that "my god is better than your god, my scripture is better than your scripture." Terror at the testosterone-fueled warring nature of us humans that has been the midwife of these ancient religions and these ancient texts—religions and texts that can be the pretext for our own destruction.

CHAPTER 20

Our Own Personal Battles and Reconciliations—A Modern War and Peace

"... ideas ... both when they are right and when they are wrong, are more powerful than is commonly understood. Indeed the world is ruled by little else ... soon or late, it is ideas, not vested interests, which are dangerous for good or evil."

—John Maynard Keynes

"Science without religion is lame; religion without science is blind."

—Albert Einstein

If a little knowledge is a dangerous thing, then indeed more than a little sense of danger is a knowledgeable thing. We cannot afford to ignore the potential self-destructiveness of the human species, the willingness of any of us to cut off our noses to spite our faces, especially in our service to the god of our fathers. Irrational groupthink can consume us. With our current capabilities for mass slaughter— this way for the gas, ladies and gentlemen; this way for the planes used as missiles; this way for the nuclear bombardments—we cannot afford to allow our religions to be agents and catalysts for this self-destruction.

The history of the Aztec culture in Central America offers a cautionary tale, as described by Nicholas Wade. In developing a horrific set of religious beliefs, the Aztecs rose to power seven hundred years ago. But in those religious beliefs were also the seeds for their own destruction, not just the seeds for power and wealth. Using a tradition of human sacrifice, the Aztecs took this tradition to untold heights—with a lunatic objective of capturing as many people as possible from neighboring areas and slaughtering them, all in the bizarre belief that their patron god, the sun god, required massive amounts of human blood to renew his life force. This religious ideology created a society devoted overwhelmingly to a single goal, a drive to excel in warfare and in slaughter. This literal bloodthirstiness, this voracious appetite for human blood had one fatal flaw: Over time the Aztecs lost any semblance of a workforce to work the fields; they had killed most of their potential workers and servants. They had too many warriors and leaders and not enough basic labor, and they became easy prey for Cortes in 1519, especially with the unflagging help of neighboring tribes that reviled the Aztecs. The blessing from the sun god had become a curse; the upward curve of the wave had given way to a calamitous downward arc.

The Aztecs had desperately needed someone, some influential small group in their midst, to question their basic religious assumptions—to find a way out of the morass they were creating for themselves, to alter a religious ideology that was inevitably leading to their own destruction. To dehypnotize themselves, to take themselves out of their sun-god trance.

Yes, free will and necessity can coexist. Yes, the waves we are riding seem to have a certain inevitability. And yet, we can change these wave patterns—narrow them or widen them—that otherwise seem so very predetermined. Yes, the electrons and photons are precisely where we expect them to be most of the time, but not all of the time.

Ultimately adrenaline may be able to trump testosterone. Terror, and the adrenaline that accompanies and mediates terror, can override our warring nature fueled by androgens. Fear and our adrenaline-infused terror and our amygdalan reactivity can reshape the waves. We can muster our sympathetic nervous systems to alter the testosterone-driven waves, to ride a new wave of the masculine to the feminine and eventually back to a new version of the masculine, to alter our perceptions of the gods, and to bring our views of the gods more in-line with science and more in-line with our current understanding of the universe. Our adrenaline can indeed subdue our androgens.

It is time to dehypnotize ourselves, to remove ourselves from the trance of the Abrahamic faiths. It is time to direct and muster our fears toward the literalists, the fundamentalists—those among us who believe the books of the Abrahamic faiths were written by prophets and spirits and angels all emanating from one god. It is time to direct and muster our fears toward the so-called great books, the scriptures, the sacred texts themselves. No longer can they demand devotion, no longer can they demand diligent teaching of them to our children, no longer can they demand that we worship and serve and die for a venal and vindictive god, a narcissistic and punitive god. The texts are merely historical artifacts, harking back to a time of naivete and innocence and constant warfare— all reflecting an unnuanced and unambiguous view of the world, a world of black and white, of good and evil, of believers and unbelievers.

Who could have imagined large airplanes being turned into deadly missiles on 9/11? And who could have imagined that the sacred manuscripts could have been corrupted and perverted into texts that can inspire our own demise? Can we muster enough fear of these texts and enough fear of these views of the gods to overcome our fears of the unfamiliar, our fears of change—to be able to alter our collective inner lives, to alter our collective religious and spiritual beliefs?

No need to get rid of the ancient texts. We are not talking about the banning of books, the censorship of books, the burning of books, the outlawing of books. These old scriptures contain some inspiring stories, some useful stories—stories that can teach us useful values—and some not so useful stories that teach inappropriate and bizarre and psychologically inaccurate lessons on things like masturbation and homosexuality.

Let's also separate these books from the supposed gods that wrote them or inspired them. Enough of the supposed prophets and spirits and angels and even gerunds that helped write these books. With the invention of the printing press, with the creation of film and television, with the innovation of the internet, we have almost infinitely more stories—fiction and nonfiction, all more strikingly told, and told without the pretense of being divinely inspired—to invigorate us, to teach us values, to instruct us on how to live.

And, yet, religion and spirituality have a place in our lives, a different place, perhaps, than in the previous two to three millennia. If we continue to use religion as a way of inspiring us in battle, as a way of helping us go to our deaths in warfare in service to our gods, then we are not just simply killing our enemies. We are destroying ourselves. Our nuclear capabilities, our abilities to use biological poisons, change the natural order of things. We kill ourselves and our planet in our efforts to destroy our enemies. We become modern-day Aztecs.

And, yet, we need religion to help us fight our personal battles. In the midst of these battles, we want to believe we can influence those infinitesimal lumps of energy; we want to believe we can change the place where the electron can be found on the wave. We want to believe we can communicate with and engage with the quanta to change our own personal course.

Quantum theory tells us that it is impossible to know both the position and velocity of a particle at once. When we measure the position of a particle, we disturb its velocity; when we measure the velocity of a particle, we disturb its position. Prayer and meditation can help us assess our position while changing our velocity. Likewise, prayer and meditation can help us assess our velocity while disturbing our position.

When dealing with cancers and other illnesses, when dealing with personal struggles, when facing our enemies, we may want to take a step back and measure where we are on the wave, to measure our position, to measure our velocity, to disturb our position, to disturb our velocity. We can ride the waves, *and* we can disturb the waves. Free will *and* necessity, all at the same time.

When we allow ourselves to develop a more healthy narcissism—a belief and confidence in ourselves, a narcissism in which the gods and quanta serve us, rather than vice versa—and when we allow ourselves to get rid of pathologically narcissistic gods that insist upon us serving them, we will live freer and more productive lives. No longer slaves to our gods—free at last, free at last.

When we embrace the exactitudes and inexactitudes of life, when we embrace the certainties and uncertainties of life, when we embrace the fairness and justice of life along with the unfairnesses and injustices, we will be able to die more freely, and paradoxically we will be able to live more freely.

Arguably the most compelling purpose of religion and spirituality is to help us deal with and manage death. Religious rituals for dealing with death are crucial. No need to change them. Whatever our religious background, let's hold onto these rituals; let's use these rituals to manage death, to hold onto and remember the person who has died, to internalize the significance and values of that person.

And let's hold on to our celebrations, to help us revel in life and help us repress thoughts of death. Let's hold onto Christmas, to Santa Claus, to Santeria, to festivals commemorating fall harvests—

to anything that helps us celebrate life. Let's hold onto our sacred music as well. Life without gospel music may not be a life worth living.

But let's separate these rituals and celebrations and music from the divine, from our previous conceptions of our monotheistic gods, from our books championing monotheism. Free at last, free at last.

—m—

Apoptosis—the programmed death of all living cells—may be the key to understanding life and death. The gods have set up the universe in such a way that immortality leads to mortality. Every living cell is programmed to die; every cell in the human body is programmed to die, to be replaced by a new cell that will function just as well or better than the old dying cell. When a cell, however, has a gene or protein turned off that then allows the cell to live indefinitely, cancer develops. These immortal cells reproduce and take over the body. These immortal cells take the place of the mere mortal cells. These immortal cells kill the host, kill the person, kill themselves. These immortal cells cannot live without a host—a host that they have managed to destroy.

The death of cells allows other cells to live. The death of each of us as separate human beings allows others to live. Again, a new kind of Malthusian world: We die so that others may live.

Old and stale cells that live indefinitely, old and stale organisms that live indefinitely, old and stale collective wisdoms that live indefinitely: These represent the very definition of cancer. These old and stale cells and organisms and collective wisdoms are the embodiments of a world that is unable to regenerate, to refresh itself, to redeem itself.

Only when we cling to life too ardently, only when we cling to power too ardently, only when we cling to past beliefs too ardently do we run into the accelerated death of our species. In allowing things and people and beliefs to die, we then find a way to live, to survive, to thrive. Yes, our species is programmed to die—but only by embracing our own eventual demise can we possibly extend the life of our species. Only by embracing the death of our previously cherished beliefs can we extend the life of our species. Only by embracing the contradictions and complementarities of life and death can we extend the life of our species. Only by embracing all of the current knowledge and wisdom of our society—and all its future knowledge—can we extend the life of our species.

Another transcendent paradox: The ultimate regeneration, the ultimate redemption for a cell, for an organism, for a set of beliefs is death itself. For any element of life to regenerate and refresh itself, it has to die first. Apoptosis, or programmed cell death, rules our universe. When we defy apoptosis, a cancer is inevitable.

A crucial note, a warning to atheists and agnostics: It is essential for you to make any renewal in religion and spirituality *your* business, even if you cannot believe in the quanta, in the photons, in the waves, in the gods. By dismissing this spirituality, by ignoring it, by wishing it away, by having contempt for it, you are inadvertent enablers of our current waves of fundamentalism. Not unlike many partners of alcoholics, you are ignoring and wishing away the craziness and drunken deludedness of your fellow travelers, the literalists and the fundamentalists. By putting your heads in the sand, you are allowing and enabling the craziest members of our planet to run the show. You cannot kill religions via nonreligion. The faith instinct tells us that only religion can kill religion. Yes, fight fire with fire.

And find a way to engage with religion and spirituality. Make distinctions between a religiosity that is out of control and one that is manageable and in control—not unlike the spouse of a heavy-drinking partner who has to figure whether the partner's drinking is out of control or manageable and responsible. An old Japanese proverb: first the man takes the drink, then the drink takes the drink, then the drink takes the man. Likewise, is religion taking over the man, or is the man still in control over his religion?

—⁓—

Where do religion and spirituality fit into my own life? What the hell is a nice Jewish boy doing in talking about the end of the monotheism of his ancestors? For that matter, what was a nice Jewish boy doing in the surgical amphitheater of Columbia-Presbyterian Medical Center in New York City, anesthetized and having his pelvis torn apart on Yom Kippur day, October 5, 1984?

I simply wanted to figure out where I fit into, and where our species and our planet fit into, the universe. Why do we live? Why do we die? Why do bad things happen to seemingly good people? Why do good things happen to apparently bad people? Why do drunken drivers have the right of way? Are we merely sheep being fattened up for the slaughter?

Religion and spirituality are an effort to motivate ourselves in the midst of a battle, to inspire us, to help us face death, and to also face life. I have faced a remarkable foe in the form of prostate cancer. It has put up an exceptional battle; I have fought gamely as well. If it—this prostate cancer—does not win the battle, something else will kill me instead.

Our battles can now become more personal, more individualized— sometimes, but not necessarily, community versus community, nation versus nation, region versus region, religion versus religion, ethnic tribe versus ethnic tribe, one -ism versus another ism. "He who conquers men has force, he who conquers himself is truly strong," notes Lao Tse. I wish to have force *and* strength. I want to live with death and battle death. I want to live with prostate cancer and battle prostate cancer. I want to live with myself and battle myself. My cancer is me, and my cancer is not me.

I wish to have a dialogue with the gods, with the quanta. I wish to give in to them and disturb them, to live with them and change them. I want a religious and spiritual perspective that helps me go into battle but not into battle necessarily with my enemies— instead, into a battle with disease, a battle with dying, a battle with death.

I have no trouble with the military metaphors attached to cancer, despite the protestations of Susan Sontag in *Illness as Metaphor*. Yes, cancer is malignant and deadly. Yes, cancer is invasive. It infiltrates; it consumes; it takes over. It refuses to die; it only dies when it has killed the host organism. Yes, cancer kills, and cancer kills itself.

So, I have no trouble with the notion of trying to kill and eviscerate and torch and nuke cancer cells. The cancer and I are in arched battle. I will use desperate and drastic measures to destroy this disease. "Diseases desperate grown by desperate appliance are relieved, or not at all," Shakespeare reminds us. I will use nuclear force and poisons, not on my enemies, but on myself and on my own cells that otherwise refuse to die. I will use my dialogue with the gods, the quanta, to motivate me and mobilize me into battle. I will engage in my own war on cancer.

We now have a way to channel our warlike natures—to turn our bellicosity and our warring impulses toward our own internal adversaries, toward our own genetic faults. We can battle against death and at the same time give in to death. Dying is as natural as living. None of us has to make any extra effort to die. We do not have to torch and nuke the planet. Like all of us, the planet can die its own natural death—without our assistance.

I will fight the gods, or the quanta, and yet give in to the quanta. I will pray to the gods, to the quanta, to alter the path of these unseeable lumps of energy. I will make every effort to modify the wave I am riding, to shift its path, to reshape the arc of any downward curves, to alter my position and my velocity in this downward arc.

At the same time I will give in to the natural trajectory of life and death when the quanta follow the expected path, when I am facing the ultimate point in that downward arc—death itself.

Religion and faith and spirituality will always be with us. There is indeed a faith instinct, a religion impulse. Faith helps us go into battle, it helps us face illness and death, it helps us deal with the finiteness of life, it helps us try to figure out what happens after we die. So, I want to have faith—to have faith in the gods, in the quanta, in those infinitesimal lumps of energy, in those waves that are also particles. I want to face death with the assistance of these gods, these quanta.

A belief in the gods helps us to care less, to take the pressure off. No wonder athletes get together in a prayer circle before a major sporting event: It is all in the hands of the gods; it is beyond my control. I will do my best in this pursuit, but so much of life—so much of what happens in this sporting event or in life itself—is predetermined, is outside of my control. With the help of the gods, we move from the land of "choke"—the pressure to perform is overwhelming—to a point in which the stress level is manageable, to a point in which we can care less. With a belief that the gods, the quanta, the photons, are with us, we can care less. We can then function and perform at an optimal level.

Whether facing an athletic contest or an illness or death, we can perform more effectively if we believe the gods are with us. We are not alone in this struggle. We can believe in the waves we are riding; we can let these waves take their course, without our trying too hard, without our pressuring ourselves too hard, without our working too hard to change these wave functions. We can fight loss and death, yet give in to loss and death at the same time. We can care about the outcome and at the same time care less.

Let us not underestimate how crucial faith and religion can be for anyone who has grown up with punitive parenting, or with no parenting at all. A faith in the gods gives us another chance to be reparented—to project onto the gods a positive and caring presence that can provide a corrective emotional experience. As long as we can avoid any negative transference projections—the tendency to project onto the gods our negative and punitive experiences with parents and other authority figures—the gods in all their projected glorious positivity can help us become loving and caring partners and parents and work colleagues and friends.

And let us not underestimate the value of a higher power in taking us away from forces like drugs and alcohol—from anything that has taken power over us, that has come to control our lives. We human beings instinctually need a sense that there is a power larger than ourselves, a power larger than drugs or alcohol, a power larger than cancer and disease, a power larger than life and death. As Bill W. and Dr. Bob have pointed out, it is invaluable to admit we are powerless, to be able to turn ourselves over to a higher power. The power of paradox: only with our acknowledgement of our powerlessness and helplessness do we gain power and liberation and control.

And let us not underestimate the value of the religious impulse in helping us channel our obsessiveness and compulsiveness and superstitiousness. In the face of doubt and uncertainty and ambiguity, we have an inherent desire and need to reestablish some semblance of control. "If I do this or that, something good will happen; the gods will look favorably upon me." Rain will come; health will come; victory over my adversaries will come; wealth will come. These beliefs and rituals are essential for our survival.

A paraphrasing of the third step in Alcoholics Anonymous (A.A.) is vital as we move into the twenty-first century—to turn our will and our lives over to the care of gods as we understand them. Bill W. and Dr. Bob got it right. Our understanding of God or gods can evolve; our understanding of the gods and the universe is not static; our understanding of our planet does not remain stagnant and stale over the course of twenty-five hundred years. Our universe expands and evolves, our species expands and evolves, and our understanding of the gods expands and evolves.

—⁂—

Is it lights-out when we die? The big sleep, the eternal sleep? Sukie Miller, a therapist who has studied how people think of death in various cultures, has noted that it is easier to die if we have a picture in our minds—coherent or incoherent, rational or irrational, it does not matter—of what happens in the after-death.

Some elements of the after-death seem obvious to many of us: We do not remain full-bodied organisms that rise into the heavens or descend into the netherworld. We do not come back as other people or other species, plant or animal. Men do not find themselves in a blissful setting in which they are cavorting with seventy-two virgins. All of these are pleasant ideas that make death more palatable than it really is.

Here's my view—just as incoherent and irrational as any other view: We remain part of the quanta, we are lumps of energy, we continue to be waves and particles, affecting other waves and other particles—with no capacity for consciousness, no human or earthly capabilities. Whether we have been buried or burned after we die, we are still spirits and energies and qi—whatever name you wish to apply to it—that remain in the universe, still to be felt and experienced by people left behind. We do not have eyes or brains; we do not look down from above; we are not anthropomorphic entities watching our loved-ones' every move. As if in a thought experiment a la Erwin Schroedinger and Albert Einstein, we are alive and dead at the same time, we have an impact here and there and everywhere— here on earth and on energy and particles perhaps millions of light-years away.

In the meantime, as long as we remain alive, all we can do is remain vigilant, to recognize and observe and measure the malignancies among us—and to eliminate them if at all possible, or to find a way to keep them in check, or to manage to live with them if necessary. We can excise them; we can nuke them; we can poison them; we can even castrate them—anything we can do to reprogram cells and organisms to die and not live indefinitely. We can find a way to deal with the malignancies among us—malignancies that are grossly unaware of their own malignant nature.

All I can do, with my prostate cancer and with any other limitations and infirmities that come along, is maintain my commitment to what Saul Bellow once bellowed, "that freedom to approach the marvelous which cannot be taken from us, the right, with grace, to make the most of what we have." Or, as Tolstoy once extolled, "to love life in all its countless, inexhaustible manifestations." To exult in the cockeyed cavalcade of life.

I will follow the lead of that silver-tongued and silver-haired devil, Jimmy Dale Gilmore, the only singer-songwriter I know of who enjoys the whim of combining quantum physics with Buddhist teachings. Here is what my particles as waves are doing:

Tonight I think I'm gonna go downtown,
Tonight I think I'm gonna look around,
For something I couldn't see when this world was more real to me,
Tonight I think I'm gonna go downtown.

Whether dead or alive, we will all be going downtown and uptown at the same time. We will be going in all directions at once. Downtown, then uptown, then across town, from in-town to out-of-town, then from out-of-town to in-town, from the real to the unreal, from the unreal to the real. We are filled with infinite quanta; we follow infinite pathways. Keep riding the waves, keep disturbing the waves, keep enjoying the ride . . .

CHAPTER 21

The Wonders of Irony and Paradox and Ambiguity

"The only thing that makes life possible is permanent, intolerable uncertainty; not knowing what comes next."
—Ursula LeGuin

"It is not so much that there are ironies of history, it is that history itself is ironic. It is not that there are no certainties, it is that it is an absolute certainty that there are no certainties."
—Christopher Hitchens, *Hitch-22*

The purposefully ambiguous life. In facing the snares of prostate cancer, I became a world-class expert in dealing with ambiguity. No certitudes, no algorithms, no sureties. Flying by the seat of my pants.

I was dealing with the first sign of a visible and palpable metastasis. It was May 2004, twenty years after my initial diagnosis, twenty years after surgery and radiation, fifteen years after my first clear-cut rise in the PSA, fifteen years after the first signs of invisible metastatic disease. I had been waiting for this day: Eventually the cancer will latch onto bone, spread into my lymph nodes, become visible. It has been lurking for two decades—ready to pounce.

For the thirteen years since going on the intermittent androgen blockade, I had scanned my body whenever the PSA had risen to eight—just before I re-induced the chemical castration. No signs of visible disease until now. Bone scans had been normal even though prostate cancer is notorious for spreading into the bone before locating itself anywhere else. CT scans had also shown no signs of disease.

In May 2004, the bone scan was again normal. We physicians call this bone scan "negative"—meaning it is negative for any apparent disease—even though for the patient a negative bone scan is anything but negative. A sigh of relief—until I saw the CT scan of my chest. Although there was no sign of spread to my lymph nodes, there was a highly suspicious mass in my right lung. Not rounded, having rough edges, it was not a benign granuloma. This was a tumor mass—a cancerous mass, albeit relatively small.

I heard a unified chorus. "Prostate cancer never goes to the lungs, especially in its first-ever metastasis," said some prostate cancer experts whom my internist consulted with.

"You have some kind of primary lung cancer until proven otherwise," said a thoracic surgeon. Helen and I were sitting in his mahogany-walled office in downtown Washington, DC. He was looking at the CT scan. "This tumor is rather inaccessible. Not many surgeons can get to it. I am one of the few who can do it safely."

This guy's confidence was breathtaking.

Yet his reasoning and decision-making may have been half-baked. I did not doubt he had great hands, that he might be among the best at getting to inaccessible lung lesions. Did I want him, though, breaking a few ribs and splaying my lungs all over an operating table if the tumor was prostate cancer?

Ah, "the wisdom of crowds." I now had a phrase to describe what I had been doing for the past fifteen years. I refused to rely on one single expert. I called the Gerald Murphys, the Nicholas Bruchovskys. I consulted with experts from all over the US, from Canada, from different medical specialities—conventional experts, eccentric experts. My job was to aggregate the divergent opinions. Who could do it better than the person whose life was at stake?

I had just read James Surowiecki's *The Wisdom of Crowds: Why the Many Are Smarter Than the Few and How Collective Wisdom Shapes Business, Economies, Societies and Nations.* And how collective wisdom was shaping my own medical decision-making.

Yes, a group of independent and diverse and decentralized experts comes up with the wisest decision more often than almost any one individual. No need to get caught up in an echo chamber, in a point of view in one institution, in one part of the country, that has taken on a life of its own—a point of view that can no longer be debated and contradicted.

This apparent cancer in my right lung became a Rorschach card, a set of ink blots, onto which any expert could project his or her own form of optimism or pessimism. Their perspective told me as much about them and their way of thinking as it did about the actual tumor.

Some experts echoed what the thoracic surgeon had just told me, "You've probably got a rapidly growing lung cancer, not prostate cancer. We've got to get in there, biopsy it, remove it as soon as possible. Your life is in major danger."

Others seemed to be overly optimistic, "It's probably nothing. Sure, your PSA is rising again. But you can just watch and wait and see what happens."

But then a consensus emerged. "Simply go back on the androgen blockade. Your PSA will head back toward zero. And if this tumor is actually prostate cancer, the tumor will recede, it will shrink. If it is a primary lung cancer—a new separate cancer that has started in your lungs—the tumor will grow larger and expand. If it is a benign granuloma—its rough edges, though, make it look like anything but a benign lesion—it will not change much at all."

Who knew that a crowd of experts could come up with a simple but elegant game plan? A game plan, though, that was filled with ambiguity and uncertainty.

I was beginning to realize that many of the experts I was consulting had more trouble dealing with ambiguity and uncertainty than I did. Yes, I did want answers just as any human being does. Yes, I did want to know what this tumor was made of. Yes, I did know that prostate cancer seldom went into the lungs in its initial foray into the land of metastases. Yes, I did know I was taking a gamble: If the tumor turned out to be a rapidly growing new lung cancer, I had waited a bit too long to intervene.

But chill out, guys. I am the one taking the risks, not you all. It all comes back to the psyche. Can I shore up my psyche? Can I shore up my ability to live with ambiguity and uncertainty? And can I help you guys live with this uncertainty as well?

Yes, uncertainty is risk that is tough if not impossible to measure—risk that is virtually incalculable, risk that has few if any precedents. Unlike a blackjack hand where one can calculate the actual risk, where one can calculate the risk, say, in doubling down or in splitting eights, I was dealing with what Nate Silver calls a "back-of-the-envelope estimate (of risk) that may be off by a factor of 100 or by a factor of 1,000; there is no good way to know."

Yes, how could *I* chill out?

—m—

The answer about the tumor came within a few weeks. The PSA had dropped steadily, and a new CT scan showed a rapidly receding tumor. The new consensus: Prostate cancer gets funky after sitting in your body for twenty years. This two-decade-old disease had found some nice little niches after all these years.

With the help of my internist, I consulted with a different thoracic surgeon. Should we still be looking at the possibility of surgically removing this one and only metastasis, especially now that it was shrinking?

This surgeon ended up defying all stereotypes, the notion that surgeons cut, boxers box, psychiatrists say, "Uh, huh," all day.

She took a quick look at the films and asserted, "You don't need me, you don't need a surgeon. We can get this thing radiated. You'll be as good as new."

No muss, no fuss—no blood, no gore, no breaking of ribs, no destruction of muscle and soft tissue. No major collateral damage.

Georgetown University had a new cyberknife, the surgeon pointed out, a piece of equipment that delivered radiation in a more focused and localized and efficient way. Instead of my needing to come in for a couple of minutes of radiation treatment every day for six weeks—as I had done in early 1985 for radiation to the prostate bed—I now only had to come in for three days, or five days, for thirty-five to forty-five minutes a shot.

Ah, there is no accounting for the inventions that John Maynard Keynes imagined as changing the economy, a society, our world—and now changing my world of well-being. Breakthroughs are breaking through.

A few metal markers placed into my right lung to establish the location of the metastasis, throw in a bit of castration—getting my PSA as close to zero as possible—to make the cancer cells as vulnerable to radiation as possible. And then the radiation itself over a three day period in February 2005.

Voila—the tumor has disappeared, never to return to that specific location again.

—∞—

The disappearance of the tumor did not quite drown out a unified chorus. I continued to hear, "You have had your first of perhaps many ongoing visible metastases. It is now time to bite the bullet, to stay on the androgen blockade for the rest of your life." Chemical castration had replaced surgical castration over the past twenty years. Surgical castration is irreversible; chemical castration is reversible—but the two interventions might as well be one and the same.

"Stay the course. Do not reverse course. If this treatment is working, why change anything? Why go off the medication? Why would you consider not being castrate?" Huh? Why would I consider being castrate the rest of my life, if it is not absolutely necessary?

I still had Gerald Murphy's voice ringing in my head, and I still had Nick Bruchovsky literally speaking in my ear.

Nick continued to remind me: If you stay on the androgen deprivation treatment for too long, the cancer cells will find another substance to fuel their growth. They will no longer need testosterone to stimulate them. Treatment will then become much trickier. You have a cancer that is hormone sensitive and radiation sensitive. Let's take full advantage of those elements for as long as we can.

Yes, less is more. A tricky concept to get across. $2 > 5$. None of this computed for many of the physicians I was consulting with. I at least had had fifteen years to let it begin to compute.

—⁂—

The final piece in the polishing of the brains of each of us: in late adolescence and young adulthood, and no earlier, we develop a capacity to handle ambiguity and uncertainty, and all the frustrations that come with the crazy bounces and nuances of life.

In very early childhood, we are programmed as a species for language development. We are sponges at the age of two or three, picking up words and syntax and grammar of any language we are exposed to. Then comes mathematics in our first years of schooling, during the so-called latency years. Scientific thinking and abstract reasoning become more assured at the age of eleven and beyond. Throughout our childhoods and adolescences, we are ingrained with the rules of a society—the spoken and unspoken rules. Everything is clear-cut, cut and dry, black and white. The answers are incontestable and indisputable: 1+1=2, 5 > 2; the Earth revolves around the sun; one inch equals 2.54 centimeters; killing someone is illegal except in the context of war.

Then come the gray areas. We begin to refine and polish our brains. Nuances seem to appear everywhere. Skepticism and even cynicism—all of which can turn into bitterness under the wrong circumstances later in life—rear their head. Do I believe in the god I have been taught to believe in? Do I believe in the religion of my forefathers? How do I make sense of life and death? How do I face the ambiguities of living and dying?

Arguably young adults can handle ambiguity and uncertainty better than older adults. This ambiguity is new to them, a fresh challenge. The stakes are not nearly as high as for older adults: Death does not feel imminent. That wonderful sense of immortality gives us a sense we can face anything. Nothing is off-limits, nothing is sacred. We can talk and joke about anything, including sex and god and death and destruction—and all their nuances.

Our ability to handle ambiguity and nuances may not last long.

As we get older, we get scared. The stakes are too high. We have kids; we sense their vulnerability; we recognize our own fragility. We get frightened of our own thoughts, and we want to perish certain thoughts—because of the irrational fear that thoughts and ideas can lead to calamity. Long before we are sans teeth, sans eyes, sans taste, sans everything, we are without the courage, without the appetite, to fully face the ambiguities of life. We desperately look for certitudes. We bargain with the gods: If I am a good god-fearing person, I will be spared, I will be saved, I will survive and thrive. We lose our ability to challenge the gods, to see that much of life is a joke, to retain our skepticism and cynicism. We can regress to concreteness; we can give up our ability to manage ambiguity and abstractions.

In science the best way to study a specific brain function is to study its loss. We now know the areas of the brain that are involved in language development, in vision, in memory, in emotion, and in handling stress—all learned from people who have lost these capacities from accidents, strokes, and surgeries. The capacity to handle ambiguity is subtler, but we now have been able to observe human beings—and even laboratory rats—who have been unable to develop this capacity to handle nuances, whose subtle development of cognitive flexibility has been stunted.

We now have data on adults who began binge drinking in early to mid-adolescence and continued this binge drinking for ten or twenty years. Their forebrains—specifically the orbitofrontal cortex, which uses associative information to envision future outcomes—can be significantly damaged by binge drinking. With this cortical damage, even after years of sobriety, these former or current binge drinkers can fail to recognize the consequences of their actions. Their ability to make wise decisions, to recognize the impact of these decisions, to change course if necessary, is compromised.

Studies on lab rats confirm these findings. At the University of North Carolina Bowles Center for Alcohol Studies, researchers placed two groups of rats into large tubs of water. The rats were forced to swim around until they found a platform on which to stand—or else drown. One group contained rats that were exposed to and drank large amounts of alcohol during their adolescent and young adult years and then had the alcohol withdrawn for a number of rat-years—an enforced sobriety during a large part of their adult life. The other group—the controls—were never exposed to alcohol. They were lifelong teetotalers.

Both groups found the platform equally well, equally quickly. But when the platform was moved, the recovering alcoholic rats almost drowned. They kept circling the old location of the platform. They stayed the course.

The teetotaling control group had no such trouble.

Fulton Crews at the University of North Carolina has shown that binge drinking in rats diminishes the genesis of nerve cells; it shrinks the development of the branchlike connections between brain cells and contributes to neuronal cell death. The binges activate an inflammatory response in rat brains especially in the hippocampus. Even after long-standing sobriety, this inflammatory response translates into an exaggerated tendency to stay the course, a diminished capacity for relearning, along with maladaptive decision-making. All this occurs without any real change in what we consider "intelligence."

In the human brain, according to Dr. Crews, the cingulate cortex shows signs of neuro-inflammation after repeated alcohol binges. Our ability to adapt when the goalposts have been moved diminishes.

A cautionary tale for all of us.

—m—

So, how do we maintain our ability to embrace ambiguity, to nuzzle with nuance?

Prostate cancer and its metastases will do the trick.

In October 2006, with my PSA rising while off treatment, while noncastrate, we found on my CT scan a lymph node in my mediastinum (the upper chest, just under the sternum) that was enlarged and probably cancerous. A few weeks later the thoracic surgeon who had previously referred me for cyberknife radiation removed the lymph node along with a smaller adjacent node. The enlarged node was indeed filled with prostate cancer cells, no doubt trucked over from the prior lung lesion. The lymphatic system and its nodes provided a drainage system for these foreign cancer cells. We now, however, had more definitive proof that the lung lesion, radiated but unbiopsied, was an actual prostate cancer metastasis. Ambiguity gave way to certitude, albeit two years later.

The second node was perfectly normal, with no sign of cancer.

No rest for the weary, however. Six months later, with the PSA rising appropriately after going off treatment—we wanted the PSA to rise when testosterone was reintroduced into my system, as a sign that the cancer was still sensitive to androgens—we found another metastasis in my left rear skull. Radiation over a five-day period a few months later cleared it, especially with the cancer cells more fragile and vulnerable when I was on treatment—indeed castrated. The PSA returned to close to zero. These cancer cells remained radiation-sensitive and hormone-sensitive.

Two years later in November 2008, another mediastinal lymph node was found and quickly removed. This time the margins of the node were not clear; cancer cells appeared to have extended beyond the border of the node into the tissue outside of the node, the muscle and fascia. So, another round of the cyberknife—radiation to the right mediastinum to eliminate any of those errant cancer cells and bring them to justice.

—ᴍ—

Prostate cancer has become a literal game. Is it an old video game, a Pac-Man trek? Am I going after space invaders or asteroids? Am I in a carnival shooting arcade? Those damn elusive pellets, they keep reversing directions, showing up in weird places, invading spaces, and gaining on me. Should I reverse course? Should I stay the course? These pac-dots seem to have a mind of their own; they are brilliant in their ability to maneuver, to find a way to survive despite my best efforts to gobble them up.

A more than worthy opponent. I yearn for the day I can shake their hand and say, "Nice game. We'll meet again toward the end of the season. Or, we'll meet again in the playoffs. Or, we'll meet again next season."

But there is no end of the season. There are no final playoffs. There is no next season. The game is endless. Endless, at least until the monsters beat me and kill me. The game is fixed. We know who is going to win. We know who is the ultimate gobbler.

But I cannot stop my own gobbling. I keep at it compulsively and assertively and passionately. Gobbler versus gobbler. I want to shake my enemies by the scruff of the neck and remind them that if they win the game and kill me, they lose. They die too. It is the ultimate lose-lose game. Let's call a truce. Bug off, stop the treadmill. But this is an idiotic opponent, an opponent that has no idea about the consequences of its actions, no idea that by winning it is losing, and that by living and thriving it is dying. I cannot talk any sense into it. It has its own moronic compulsiveness, its own instinctive aggressiveness.

So, I kept gobbling whenever I found a new set of pellets. Another skull lesion, probably some rogue cells from the previous skull metastasis in the left parietal-occipital area, was discovered in December 2009. At the same time, a small metastasis was found in the thoracic spine—the T8 vertebra, to be exact.

We gobbled up the cells in both spots with the cyberknife in February and March 2010.

Those fuckers, those pellets, those Aztecs, really know how to hurt a guy. A worthy opponent, yes, but also a mean and nasty opponent. In mid-January, 2011, we found a small metastasis in my brain, in the periphery of my left parietal-occipital region, perhaps again due to some rogue cells not fully killed by the prior radiation treatments to the adjacent skull. Now they were causing real damage—some swelling and edema in that area of the brain.

This game was getting serious. The fuckers were hitting me where I made my living. I worked with my brain, with my central nervous system, to help others manage their brains and their nervous systems. I was now the wounded healer, *not* a wounded healer who is truly wounded, a wounded healer unable to heal himself, let alone others.

I could now sense the terror my physicians were feeling on my behalf. I was feeling it too. The headaches were brutal—I could sympathize with anyone having severe, or even modest, migraines.

But, voila, within a week after returning to androgen-deprivation, the treatment began to work again. Like magic, the cells went into retreat. The headaches resolved. Prostate cancer or brain cancer, as a simple head cold, metastatic prostate cancer as a simple one-week flu, prostate cancer as a simple gastrointestinal bug. The body and brain recovered quickly. A thing of beauty. Who could have imagined the inventions of the late twentieth and early twenty-first century? Thank you, Dr. Huggins and Hodges, those 1966 Nobel Prize winners for discovering testosterone as the fuel for prostate cancer growth. Thank you, Nick Bruchovsky, for discovering that less castration is better than more.

Five months later, with the PSA close to zero and the cancer cells at their nadir in strength, I got the brain metastasis radiated. There were no signs of any recurrence in the brain four years later.

But, whoa. Prostate cancer metastasizing to the brain: Was this not a sign of a terribly aggressive disease? Was this not a sign that you must become castrate for the rest of your life? So said a chorus of physicians I consulted with.

Yet there was an equally strong chorus telling me to continue the treatment protocol that worked effectively now for twenty-three years. It was still working. The spread of the cancer to the skull and now to the brain represented old disease, twenty-seven-year-old disease that went back to 1984. Before the advent of PSAs, before the advent of easy scanning, men would come into a hospital with prostate cancer everywhere, in their bones, their lungs, their brains. These men had undiagnosed disease that had been messing with them for ten to twenty years without realizing it. The difference here was that I had been more than aware; I had been watching it, scanning it, discovering it, fighting it. Old disease has a way of going wherever it pleases. After more than twenty years, it knows where the best nooks are to hang out. It knows where to find a home.

Computer simulations of my cancer, done by some colleagues of Nick Bruchovsky in Japan, indicated that the cancer cells were still mostly hormone-sensitive. Over time some hormone-insensitive cells evolved. No surprise there. But by doing the treatments intermittently, I might be able to retain a maximum level of hormone sensitivity for a maximum period of time.

Game on. You bastard pellets, make my day. Go to my brain, go wherever you please. You have long ago gone to my pelvis, my penis, my brain, and in my midsection. You have intermittently castrated me, anguished me, created catastrophe for me. I am still ready for you. I can still withdraw the androgens you rely on, I can still radiate you bastards.

I may at times be a shell of my former self. But who isn't? I have still been a battling shell, albeit an occasionally baffled shell. Those bastard cells have had to take me seriously, as I have taken them. Two serious opponents going at it in a serious way. There would be no tie games here, no games in which no one wins and no one loses.

I would keep scanning the game board, my body—looking for those bastard cells to poke their heads out of strange nooks. But these were oligometastases, limited metastases, only one or two at a time at most, not a whole host of them ready to knock me off. They continued to be findable, seeable, treatable. A thing of beauty.

Vigilantism has paid off. My vigilantes were the radiologists and their technicians—the CT scanners, the MRI studiers, the bone scanners. We scoured the pictures looking for an accretion of those pellets. We aimed, shot, and fired. We gulped; we gobbled. No sympathy for those devils.

So, how was I dealing with ambiguity and uncertainty? Decently, I guess. Was I staying the course too insistently? Was it time to change course—and was I unwilling to do so? Where was my cognitive flexibility? Just because something worked for twenty-three years did not mean it was the route to continue on.

All I could do was rely on the wisdom of crowds, to get input and feedback from various parts of the country, from prostate cancer cowboys and from prostate cancer traditionalists, from eccentrics and reactionaries.

Here's the rub: Even my questioning and confrontational internist had begun to believe in what I had been doing for the past two decades, to the point that he wondered, "Why would you change now? You have defied all expectations. Why would you go back to the traditional route? Do it your way."

My way? I did not have a specific way. Each new metastasis required some new rethinking. Is it time to change directions, or do I stay the course? Am I circling around the old location of the platform in a huge tub of water—with the platform nowhere to be found? Am I about to drown?

All I could do was stick to two principles: Let's keep the cancer hormone-sensitive as long as we possibly can. To be able to shrink tumors in the brain or lungs or bone in a matter of a week or two was astounding.

And let's keep using the radiation-sensitivity of the cancer as a weapon ready to be invoked at any time. Another thing of beauty: With the androgen deprivation the cancer cells become dormant, withered and half dead, ready to come alive again with the return of testosterone. With radiation the cancer cells perish, never to be seen again. Their demise, a thing of beauty.

In the meantime I tried new ideas, new courses of action. Thalidomide, but no effect. Then Revlimid, a derivative of Thalidomide, but no effect. Wonderful in theory: The idea was to prevent the arms and legs of those fetal and undifferentiated prostate cancer cells from growing, to immobilize those cells and kill them off. Thalidomide had been used as a sleeping pill in the 1950s until it was recognized as a drug that caused horrific congenital teratogenesis—malformations to the arms, legs, eyes, ears, and heart in a developing fetus. We now know that Thalidomide blocks the development of blood vessels and angiogenesis so that limbs and organs cannot develop properly.

All Thalidomide did for me was put me to sleep. A fine sleeping pill. But it did not stop the rise in PSA when I was off the hormonal blockade, nor did it stop the development of the occasional metastasis.

In June 2007, a few months after my first bony metastasis had been found, an oncologist recommended I try an intravenous injection of zoledronic acid, otherwise known as Zometa. A new bisphosphonate known to shore up and strengthen bone, this drug showed some promise in preventing bony metastases in breast cancer. Why not give it a try with prostate cancer?

A disaster for me. Within forty-eight hours I developed a flu-like syndrome that lasted for months. Fatigue and muscle aches—I could barely get my head off a pillow. I was immobilized and the symptoms showed no sign of letting up.

The oncologist refused to believe that the medication could have caused this syndrome. "It must be a return of your cancer; you must have a spread of prostate cancer throughout your body. You have cancer-induced cachexia." She did not have to explain this term. My PSA was close to zero, but she was convinced that I had a wildly spreading prostate cancer that was now suddenly end-stage, causing a profound loss of energy and my impending death. She insisted I get more scans to prove her point. She was ready to put me into hospice care.

Her logic was baffling. My PSA was virtually zero. I had just had an injection of some new medication whose side effects were not well-known. I had no choice but to become my own doctor again.

I called the editors of *The Medical Letter*, a biweekly four-page newsletter about pharmacology that I had been subscribing to since medical school. They kindly gave me the names of two of their consultants who had been using Zometa experimentally and extensively to help with osteoporosis.

One of them gave me the scoop: "We've been using Zometa on older women and some men with osteoporosis here at the University of Colorado Medical Center in Denver. Medicare has designated our center as a place where we can try Zometa and get reimbursed for its use. No other place has had the extensive experience we have had with the drug. The Food and Drug Administration, the FDA, has not approved Zometa yet for osteoporosis, but the approval should be coming in the next six to twelve months (in fact the drug was subsequently approved under a new name "Reclast" specifically for osteoporosis). We'll have even more experience at that time.

"We have already had four patients who have had your flu-like syndrome. It can go on for months. The headquarters for Novartis—the drug company that makes Zometa—is located in Basel. They have seen one or two cases like yours in Switzerland.

"Your only choice is to use high doses of steroids, at least 60 mg. of Prednisone per day for an indefinite period of time."

The steroids worked; I was able to function. But a bone researcher I talked to on the phone reminded me that anything that gets into the bone will stay in the bone. The drug will leach out slowly but will stay in my bones for the rest of my life.

I had a choice: Fury vs. Fear. I chose fury. These bisphosphonates, the Colorado guy explained to me, were chemicals that were initially used to prevent soap from sticking to glass. Great for car washes, great for the bum on the street who was washing your windshield, great for the glass door of your washing machine, great for the bones of many people.

A disaster for me.

My fury was not so much focused on the reasonable experimental effort to prevent bone metastases—what the hell, give it a try. My fury was based on abandonment—a physician abandoning me when I had a brutal side effect that she refused to acknowledge. It was her unwillingness to admit that the medication could be causing this cachexia. It was her claim that this cachexia must be a bizarre zero-PSA wild spread of prostate cancer. It was her implicit insistence that I had to be my own doctor—to figure out if Zometa had a side effect of severe cachexia and what antidotes to use for this cachexia.

After all the years of dealing with prostate cancer, I had the confidence and hubris to be my own doctor. I also had the kindness of strangers—the physician at *The Medical Letter*, the consultants in Colorado and Maine whom he referred me to. I had access to steroids which I used successfully for five months, then tapered and discontinued, not without difficulty. But within eight months of the Zometa injection, I was back on the tennis and basketball courts; I was back on track.

Nothing like iatrogenic ambiguity, nothing like doctor-induced dubiousness. Will I become gun-shy and avoid new experimental efforts to deal with prostate cancer and its inevitable metastases? Will I continue to take some calculated risks? Will I have physicians who will not abandon me at the first sign of problems with these experimental efforts?

Time will tell.

—⁓—

As John Maynard Keynes once asked, what place is allowed for "non-numerical factors" in predicting the future—the inventions and breakthroughs that are entirely unpredictable? Expect the unexpected—and if you live long enough, you can see the unexpected unfolding. In prostate cancer the breakthroughs have had little or nothing to do with treatments. Yes, there have been some new wrinkles with androgen blockers, some new drugs in the pipeline that can block the effects of testosterone and dihydrotestosterone. And there are new wrinkles in how radiation can be delivered, with the cyberknife and other such tools that can deliver focused radiation with a minimum of collateral damage.

Instead, the real inventions have come in the way we now can find and diagnose tiny metastatic prostate tumors, even when the PSA is as low as 0.5. Up until recently we only had bone scans that allowed us to look for tumors in bones, but not at a highly sophisticated level, and we had CT scans to look at soft tissue, including lymph nodes and lungs and other areas of the body. If a lymph node was enlarged, we might want to biopsy it to determine the type of cells sitting in that node. Likewise the lungs: only a biopsy could tell us definitively what a lesion in the lungs might be made of, benign or cancerous tissue.

We now have new forms of carbon, specifically a radioisotope called C11 which can be put into chemicals such as acetate and choline, to form C11-acetate and C11-choline. Prostate cancers take up these chemicals—and suddenly prostate tumors light up. A C11-acetate positron-emission tomography (PET) scan can then be superimposed on the old technology, a bone scan—and one can then see which tiny lesions reflect true and definitive prostate lesions.

We can then do radiation treatment when the tumor burden is quite low. And, conceivably, we can then find a way to stay off the androgen blockade—chemical castration—for a longer period of time. This longer period of not being castrated may allow the cancer cells to remain hormone-sensitive for a more sustained period.

In December 2013, a C11-acetate scan in Phoenix, Arizona, was able to detect tiny prostate metastases in the L3 region of my spine and in my left parietal region of my skull, even with my PSA at a very low level. Within six weeks we were able to radiate the lesions with the cyberknife. The lesions—gone and kaput. All I can continue to do is be vigilant and wary.

Even more sensitive diagnostic tools are in the pipeline in Germany. In Heidelberg and Munich, the radioactive isotope Gallium 68 is being used in PET scans along with the C11 PET scans. The sensitivity of these scans and the brilliant and psychedelic images are remarkable.

Road trips to Phoenix, Arizona, as well as to Heidelberg or Munich, may be very much a part of my future.

Seeing metastatic disease at its inception, seeing disease when the tumor burden is low, seeing disease before the cancer has become widespread makes all our interventions more effective. Indeed a virtuous circle based not on better treatments but on better diagnostic tools.

—⁂—

A strange thing has happened to my inner life in the past year or two. I have lived longer than I ever could have expected. Unknowingly I had internalized those messages from physicians in 1984 that I had less than a 50 percent chance of living five years and a very small chance of living ten years. The power of negative thinking: Little did I know that these guys had done me a favor, that if I lived longer than expected I would be mindful and receptive to every added second, every added moment of my life, that I would be able, I think, to face death a bit more readily, to go a bit more quietly into the good night, given that I had been expecting to die twenty years ago, ten years ago, five years ago.

I am proud to be living on borrowed time. Every second of borrowed time is precious.

When I first went back to work in 1984 a month after surgery, a medical colleague gave me copies of Stephen Levine's books, including *Who Dies? An Investigation of Conscious Living and Conscious Dying* and *Healing Into Life and Death*. The books at the time helped me desensitize myself to death—to my own death and dying, to the life and death of everything in this universe. All I can remember from that time is the notion that every other word in each sentence seemed to be "death" or "dying" or "loss" or "grief." A great way to desensitize oneself to the ultimate fate: Die, Die, Die.

Only after thirty years of facing prostate cancer hell can I appreciate a piece of wisdom from *Who Dies?*

> Once someone asked a well-known Thai meditation master, "In this world where everything changes, where nothing remains the same, where loss and grief are inherent in our very coming into existence, how can there be any happiness? How can we find security when we see that we can't count on anything being the way we want it to be?" The teacher, looking compassionately at this fellow, held up a drinking glass which had been given to him earlier in the morning and said, "You see this goblet? For me, this glass is already broken. I enjoy it, I drink out of it. It holds my water admirably, sometimes even reflecting the sun in beautiful patterns. If I should tap it, it has a lovely ring to it. But when I put this glass on a shelf and the wind knocks it over or my elbow brushes it off the table and it falls to the ground and shatters, I say, "Of course." But when I understand that this glass is already broken, every moment with it is precious. Every moment is just as it is and nothing need be otherwise.

Stephen Levine goes on to point out that when we recognize our body is already broken, when we recognize we are already dead, "then life becomes precious and we open to it just as it is, in the moment it is occurring."

Yes, my sex life is dead at times; my penis is dead; my pelvis is dead; I am dead. When my pelvis comes back to life, it is more precious than ever. I pinch myself—I am still alive. Yet when I acknowledge I am dead, my children are dead, Helen is dead, how precious they and I become. I can live more readily with fear, with doubt, with uncertainty, with ambiguity. The worst has already happened. I am dead, and everyone I love and care about is dead.

My living with my brokenness for thirty-plus years allows me to joke about death—just like a teenager or young adult. Fuck it all, my pelvis is already broken or dead. At the same time, everything I love is more precious, more a source of delight, more a source of comedy and joy.

The treasures: Helen, my daughters who are now in their early thirties. The thirty-plus years I have survived, they have survived and thrived as well. Longevity counts a lot. Having a husband around, having daddy around—not daddy-o, not a failed daddy, not a dead daddy, even one with mythic qualities in his premature death—counts a lot. My daughters may understand the fragility of life more than most thirty-somethings.

Stephen Levine again: "Taking each teaching, each loss, each gain, each fear, each joy as it arises and experiencing it fully, life becomes workable. We are no longer 'a victim of life.'"

Levine and his wife Ondrea apparently spent a year acting as if that year was the final year of their lives. I would assume that for them everything became precious during that year—perhaps too precious.

What happens if you live thirty years as if each year is your last—without having to pretend it is your last, when that sense of its being your last year is palpable, not theoretical? What happens if each day, each birthday, each new year's celebration—the Roman calendar new year, the Chinese new year, the Jewish new year— all become precious milestones? The millennial milestone, the year 2000, becomes a particularly precious achievement. I have lived to see Y2K, and it is much more for me than a computer glitch.

Yes, precious and celebratory and comical—I have become one of the many here among us that feel life is but a joke. A precious joke, a joke I cling to, a joke I hope I can let go of when the time comes.

Who knows? When the time comes, despite my supposed desensitization after more than thirty years, I will be as terrified as anyone, distraught, confused, refusing to let go, greedy for more.

Time will tell.

—◁▷—

As a psychiatrist, am I a wounded healer or merely wounded? Perhaps only my patients can answer that question with some degree of objectivity. I *can* say that I understand the wave action of life better than ever before—that though filled with particles, we are also waves at the same time, that we are riding these waves—waves that we may or often may not have control over. Necessity versus free will—a predetermined destiny versus some control over our destiny. Somehow we can meld the two together. Go with the flow *and* alter the flow.

With every blessing there is the seed of a curse; with every curse there is the seed of a blessing, often, in the words of Winston Churchill as he was about to lose the 1945 election in Britain, a very, very "well-disguised blessing."

I can reassure my patients that, though the waves have buried them, though the undertow has submerged them, the waves may also allow them to rise again. The key is to stay alive, to try to stay upright. If you can live long enough, you can begin to feel the power of those waves, to experience the falls and the rises, to experience genuine awe at the hurricane action of the waves alongside at times the calmness of those same waves.

"Yes," I can say, "This depression or this panic or this grief can seem interminable. This severing of your children from you can seem unending. This horrific marriage can seem to have an unending impact. Yes, all *bad* things will come to an end. And, yes, all *good* things will come to an end too."

Patience, patience, patience. We are all patients, either now or in the future. My patienthood has lasted longer than most. My good fortune in finding a way to make a deadly illness into a chronic illness has allowed me to last longer than most.

"You, as my patient," I can say, "and I, as your doctor and fellow patient, are on a ride together. We will ride these waves together. We will try to change the trajectory of the waves together. We will give it our best shot."

Happy is the one who understands the nature of things, who has discovered the causes of things. With longevity comes an understanding of the nature of things. With the loss of lust and libido—with an inability to forget time and death—comes an understanding of the nature of things.

Only with longevity and time does a species have the opportunity to evolve. Even in the limited course of 150,000 years, the human species has evolved in a profound way. Even in the limited time of the past 10,000 years—with the stabilization of climate and temperatures on our planet and with the consequent domestication of animals and wheat and barley—have we as a species evolved. And just in the past millennium have we seen a gradual diminution in the level of violence and aggression in our species. We are indeed continuing to change and evolve.

Only with the longevity of my illness have I been able to evolve. A quick death of a species, a quick death of a human being—it goes without saying—prevents any evolving and growth and redemption. A quick death—circumstances in which one does *not* live with death hanging over one's head for, say, thirty or more years, circumstances in which one does *not* live with an inability to forget time and death— may not allow for a full-blown evolution, a full-blown salvation, a full-blown understanding of the nature of things. To last, to linger, to stay alive, to thrive in any way we can—even without sexual health and lust and luster—is crucial.

This is what I can pass on to my patients: We will do everything we can to understand the nature of things, to discover the causes of things, to survive as long as we can, to see the rises and falls in those waves we are riding for as long as we can.

—⁓—

How has Helen evolved over these past thirty or more years? Her initial reaction: "How could this be happening to us? None of our friends and peers are dealing with this. We are only in our mid-thirties. Our plate is not just full, it is overflowing, and not overflowing in a good way. Fertility and love and sex, and life itself, have been ravaged." The same questions as were asked by Ivan Illyich, asked though perhaps for different reasons.

Given that I could not tolerate my own self-pity, I was unable to tolerate Helen's. I provided a less than sympathetic ear. "There's a ton of pain in this world. I deal with it all the time in my office. Our contemporaries, and some who are younger than we are, are experiencing things that are as awful, or even worse, as what we are going through. I see it every day; I see it in my office every day."

What the hell am I saying? Come to my office, and you will get a sympathetic ear. Huh? Come to my home, though, and be part of my family—and you will barely get a tender and responsive ear. If your pain is different than what Helen and I are going through, you will get my compassion and support and guidance. As long as your night-side of life is distinct from my night-side of life, you will have a more than sympathetic ear.

My prostration from being prostateless prevented me from supporting Helen in her helplessness. I was unable to handle my own predicament at the time. And I could not accept and face Helen's predicament.

—⁓—

Through good fortune Helen and I have lived long enough that our peers have caught up with us—with their own struggles and tragedies, their prostate cancers and breast cancers, with their same Tolstoyan questions, "What is it all for? Why is this happening?" None of them have spent thirty or more years losing their lust, being unable to forget time and death. We are, in a sense, ahead of them; we are their beacon, their sentinel, their canary in the coal mine—a canary who has not died yet despite the absence of oxygen, despite the periodic loss of lust, a husband-and-wife set of canaries that have survived surgery and radiation and hormonal manipulation together.

So, you wanna know what it's like? We'll tell you what it's like. We'll tell you what it's all about. Is it wisdom? Is it hubris? Are Helen and I as a couple simply the walking wounded, or have we both in our own way become wounded healers? Or have we simply learned to keep walking despite our wounds?

A new kind of potency. A new kind of power and control. A new kind of understanding of the nature of things. The antithesis of helplessness. Helen, not unlike me, has taken the best shots the gods and the quanta can give her, and she is still standing: standing tall as a wife and mother, ready to give as good as she gets. Freakingly amazing—she has taken standing by her man to inimitable heights. I may have lived with prostate cancer and metastatic disease and intermittent castration for several decades, and more amazingly, she has been willing to live with all of my afflictions and stand by me for those same decades. Implausible, inconceivable, preposterous. Arguably more preposterous than standing by a man who has been repeatedly unfaithful.

And all the attention showered on me for the past thirty or more years: "How's Paul?" ask her friends and mine. "Is he okay? How's his health?" Rarely the question, "How are you doing, Helen? How are you holding up?" Yet she was the one facing the prospect of being a single parent in her mid-thirties into her forties.

At the same time, shame and self-consciousness have fallen by the wayside for both of us. Privacy? Privacy for my and our privates? Forget about it. We are not exhibitionists, yet we are not thirteen year-olds obsessed with keeping ourselves hidden and clothed.

If, as they say in Alcoholics Anonymous, "We are only as sick as our secrets," then Helen and I—despite my cancer, despite how affected by my cancer she has been—are among the healthiest on the planet.

—⚏—

During the Jewish new year, during Rosh Hashanah and Yom Kippur services, Jews around the world recite and chant a Hebrew prayer purportedly written by a German rabbi in the eleventh century, possibly written several centuries earlier in what is now Israel. For the coming year the prayer asks, "Who will live, who will die, who will die at his predestined time and who before his time; who by water and who by fire . . . who will rest and who will wander . . . who will be degraded and who will be exalted."

The notion is that one god will determine everyone's destinies and inscribe the verdicts for the coming year.

The singer-songwriter Leonard Cohen took the same prayer and put it to a poem and song in the 1970s. It begins in the same way as the original prayer, "Who by fire? Who by water?" Then, "Who in the sunshine? Who in the night time?. . . Who in your merry month of May? Who by very slow decay?"

But there is a punch-line after each verse: "And who shall I say is calling?"

Can we live with the ambiguity of not knowing who is calling, of not knowing precisely what the hell is going on? All we can say, perhaps, is what is *not* going on. It is inordinately unlikely that there is one god, or a god couple, a husband and wife god couple, or, say, seventeen gods, or a father and son and holy ghost set of gods, or a god who sends down prophets and angels and messengers and gerundives to direct us on how to live, to tell us who is among the faithful and who is an infidel.

Can we live without concrete gods, without concrete stand-ins for the gods—without our new idols: the Torahs, the Bibles, the Old and New Testaments, the Korans? Can we return to the abstract, to the intangible, to the impalpable, to the indefinite, to the ambiguous and uncertain? Can we avoid a regression to the concreteness of childhood, to the concrete thinking of a six-year-old?

Can we accept Martin Buber's notion that formal religious dogma is "the great enemy of mankind?"

Those frigging unseeable quanta, those bastard bundles of energy, those loopy lumps—both particles and waves, going everywhere and nowhere at the same time, on infinite pathways and on a single pathway at the same time. Not unlike those unseeable bastard prostate cancer cells, filled with their own bundles of energy, always lurking, always ready to pounce.

So, I can pray to the quanta, to the cancer cells; I can try to sway them. I can laugh at them and humor them. I can cry with them, despair with them. I might be able to arouse them and silence them. I can at least fuck with them. A little tit for tat, given how much those fuckers are fucking with me, with all of us, given how easily they can silence us, squelch us.

And who shall I say is calling?

A Twenty-First Century Keats

Warning: The following ode has no sexual innuendos. This ode has no sexually explicit or implicit content.

ODE TO ANDROGENS

Power! Control! You slayer, you source of testy torment
You pedophile, you rapist, you fucker without consent.
So facile with crime and abuse,
Never willing to consider a truce.
Warmonger, a monstrosity for mankind,
And even more: a horror for kids and womankind.

Yet I will be thy priest, and build a fane
To make your goodness known
When you are here the forests swell, the mountains shadow
    the plain
The brooks do fill, the barren trees go green, we never feel
    alone.

Can there be ambition, love, and poesy without thee?
What else will fill all fruit with ripeness to the core?
What can swell the gourd and plump the hazel shells?
What else can set the buds afloat on the wonderful vaginal
    floor?

Adieu, adieu—I am fucked through and through.
Without thee I am lost, and yet forever young.
Epicene, nothing ever obscene, I give up the profane.
I see creeks all crippled, all the rivers do drain.

Those droop-headed flowers abound.
Springtime for Hitler but where is the springtime for me?
Hast thou forsaken me, O Androgens?
The hormones: Estrogen, yes, but testosterone, no.
Where art thou, brooding hormones?
I am waiting . . . and waiting. Will you come back? Are you
        failing me now?
Is it Daddy-o? Is it Godot? Is it Androgen-o?

Thou wast not born for death, immortal hormone.
Hungry generations try to tread thee down.
But none of us can forget:
You are the creator of emperor and clown.

The swelling swagger, the babbling blather
The trophies, the towers of power
Joy and Beauty and Pleasure and Delight
Without thee, melancholy—no thrust in our engines,
        everything sour.
All is indolence without thee—my pulse grows less and less.
You give wings to man and help women flower.
Without thee, Love is worse than dour.

Vanish, ye hormones, into the clouds, but please, pretty
        please, return.
As you come back—gradual to be sure—
I begin to have visions of delight for the night,
For all the world, everything is set right.

When old age will this generation waste,
You dear hormone will remain both a friend and foe.
And ye will say in midst of other woe:
Beauty is hormonal fullness; hormonal fullness beauty—
That is all ye fuckers and non-fuckers need to know.

A Final Note

". . . a book can only end in one of two ways: truthfully or artfully. If it ends artfully, then it never feels quite right. It feels forced, manipulated. If it ends truthfully, then the story ends badly, in death . . . Life itself always ends badly."

- Jess Walter, *Citizen Vince*

Many of us die a quick death—a heart attack, a stroke, our heads severed in an automobile accident, whatever. Even cancers can lead to a precipitous death—think pancreatic cancer and melanoma. But for those of us with prostate cancer, we live and die on the installment plan, a slow slog of a slaying. We lose our lust and libido, then gain it back. We lose our lust for life, then gain it back. We get bone metastases and get rid of them via an androgen blockade or through radiation. We do likewise with lung metastases and even brain metastases. We go through rehearsal after rehearsal for our own deaths. We practice and practice. We face a death sentence over and over again, then we get reprieves. We escape the clutches of death, until we no longer can escape.

The lords of the kitchen normally boil the water first and then put the crabs—you can choose lobsters if you would like—into the hot steamy water. The crabs do not know what hit them; they die a quick precipitous death.

But for crabs like myself, the lords have put us into water at room temperature and *then* have turned up the heat. We recognize what is happening and we hightail out of the pot. The lords gather us up again, put us back into the pot. The water is a bit warmer now. We know we can still escape, and we do so. The next time the water is hotter still. We keep escaping—but we now know the end is nigh. But we deny the nighness.

Ah, denial—de Nile—yes, the biggest river in Africa. We make jokes about denial. We deny we're in denial. Those who die precipitously cling to their denial right up until their precipitous death. It is beyond their imagination. Not sick even for one day in my life, they say. I've got the reaper covered. He has nothing on me. I work out every day; I play tennis or basketball; I run practically every day.

For those of us dying on the installment plan, we keep managing our escapes. We keep finding escape routes, and we keep assuming that new hatches will open. It goes without saying that we live ultimately to die, but when facing the rapidly boiling water we are dying to live. Our denial of death allows us to extract every ounce of power and creativity out of every moment. No, I am not helpless. I can escape from that torrid water a third time, a sixth time. Feverish, slowed hopelessly by the heat, I still push forward; I grab the edge of the pot with my claws. I still hold out hope. I will still make my escape . . .